DROP
A SIZE
FOR LIFE

D0167951

Other titles by the same author:

Body Blitz
Carb Curfew
Drop a Size in Two Weeks Flat!

JOANNA HALL

DROP
A SIZE
FOR LIFE

FAT LOSS FAST AND FOREVER!

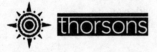

Thorsons
An Imprint of HarperCollins*Publishers*
77–85 Fulham Palace Road,
Hammersmith, London W6 8JB

The website address is: www.thorsonselement.com

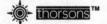 **thorsons**™

and *Thorsons* are trademarks
of HarperCollins*Publishers* Ltd

First published in 2004

4

Joanna Hall's website address is www.joannahallonline.com

Photography by Dan Welldon

A catalogue record of this book is
available from the British Library

ISBN-13   978-0-00-717527-7
ISBN-10   0-00-717527-2

Printed and bound in Great Britain by
Clays Ltd, St Ives plc

CONTENTS

INTRODUCTION

So you want to drop a size? Well, it's easy! It simply entails making some changes to your diet and stepping up your activity levels – both of which you'll learn how to do in this book. Where the real challenge lies is in maintaining that ideal size – not for a week, or a month, or even for a year, but for life.

Imagine how wonderful that would be – to achieve the body shape and size you want now and still have that figure in a decade's time. Well, you can do it – but, like most things worth having in life, it's going to take a little time, effort and know-how.

Dieting is a lot like relationships. What we're looking for in a relationship and what we're prepared to put into it influence the kind of relationship it will be. Quick-fix diets are the equivalent of a one-night stand: you get what you want fast and it feels great – but it doesn't last. You may hope for something a little more permanent but inevitably you soon realize that the man or woman of your dreams isn't all you thought they'd be and your interest wanes. Similarly, that 'revolutionary' new diet that was going to get the weight off, once and for all, soon becomes a slog and leaves you feeling disillusioned and disappointed.

Now think of a long-term relationship. Anyone who has experienced a good, lasting partnership knows that it involves a bit of work and upkeep. It's not always earth-shatteringly exciting, and there are inevitably problems along the way, but it feels right, it makes you happy and, most of all, it feels like a permanent part of your life. That doesn't mean it doesn't evolve along the way, however. More than likely, both parties change, or circumstances change, and a period of adjustment follows. The likelihood of long-term success is determined by how you navigate this sometimes tricky road.

This principle applies just as much to your relationship with your body as it does to the one you have with your partner. Things change due to circumstances, ageing, environmental and social factors, the key is to be in tune with – and responsive to – your body's needs as they arise.

Dropping a size is about weight management, not about fixing a figure on the scales and perceiving anything above that as failure. The clinical definition of successful weight management is that you stay within 20 per cent of the original weight loss. You shouldn't expect to maintain the exact same weight for life. Weight fluctuates and there are times when it is healthier to gain a little weight; times when life dictates that the effort involved in staying in shape simply can't be made. Think of it this way: if you want to stay at a weight of 9½ stones for the rest of your life, you'll need to exercise religiously and eat strictly all the time – but if you aim to stay within 20 per cent of your optimal weight, you can adopt the principles and strategies you'll learn in this book and still enjoy your life, too.

Let's go back to relationships for a moment. There are times when we think we're embarking on the ultimate relationship – 'the one' – and it turns out to be just another fly-by-night fling. At first, we can't stop thinking about our new partner, we want to talk about them all the time, we think about the future, devote loads of time to them. Then, gradually, little problems and disappointments arise, it all becomes a little mundane and we realize that they're not quite so perfect after all. Generally we carry on with the relationship a little while longer but without really giving it the care and attention it deserves to develop and improve. Inevitably a few weeks later the relationship ends – and the search for Mr Right or Mrs Right begins again.

It's a familiar enough story – but can you see how similar it is to the quest many of us are on to lose weight? Compare it to the following all-too-common scenario. You're in the coffee shop with your work colleagues and one of them tells you about this great new diet – it involves bizarre food combinations, no alcohol, no this, no that, no life but hey, it worked for Maggie in accounts and she looks fab! So you decide to leap in and really give this a go – this will be the diet for you! This diet is going to last! One month later, sitting around the same coffee table, you're back to normal eating.

That diet? Well, you lost weight initially, but you really missed your red wine and bread and you felt so devoid of energy that you couldn't possibly get to aerobics. Now you're 8 pounds heavier than when you started and a whole dress size bigger. At this point, Maggie from accounts walks past and she's most definitely gained at least two dress sizes. Ah, well, you've heard the Brussels sprouts diet is very good …

Sometimes what we think is the right diet, or the perfect relationship, really isn't. When it comes to relationships, okay we can't help it if we fall for the wrong person, or misjudge someone – and hey, we all make mistakes – but as we get older we hopefully learn from our mistakes and begin making better judgements, putting in the right kind of time and effort to the relationships that really could work. So why can't we seem to do the same with dieting? Many of us just seem to keep making the same mistakes over and over again. We keep choosing these 'Mr Right' diets and when we can't make them work we feel more and more despondent.

This repeated cycle of failure creates self-fulfilling prophecies. In other words, because you've failed before, you expect to fail again right from the outset, so you embark on your weight loss regime with 'I bet this doesn't work' in the back of your mind. With this mindset, failure is hardly surprising – and of course having proved that you are a failure, your self-esteem and confidence are further undermined.

This can actually have a negative effect on how you see yourself – on your body image. Research has shown that women who have low self-esteem have a less accurate picture of what their bodies look like than women who are more confident about themselves. Unfailingly, the under-confident women see themselves as larger than they are in reality. So not only does repeating the same mistakes fail to produce results, it may also make you feel worse than you did at the start of the whole process!

Dropping a size for life is about putting an end to this negative cycle of behaviour. This involves learning how to target your efforts to where they'll really count and about forging and nurturing a positive relationship between your body and your brain. Losing weight isn't physically hard. You know what you have to do – eat less and exercise more! However, to keep that weight off, you will need to learn how to develop mental strategies and the right mindset so that you can tackle all the challenges that life throws at us – whether it's life stages such as pregnancy, the physical effects of growing older, dealing with different emotional situations, or coping with all those everyday crises that seem to be an integral part of life in the 21st century.

GETTING STARTED

WHAT IS THE RIGHT SIZE?

The old adage 'you can never be too rich or too thin' is one that is held in much too high a regard in our society. Of course you can be too thin and striving for a size that is not realistically achievable is not only a soul-destroying business, it's also a dangerous game. You're dicing with your health and are at risk of developing disordered eating behaviours or even a full-blown eating disorder.

So what is the right size? Well judging from a recent survey, which revealed that 63 per cent of people lie about their weight, with 22 per cent not even telling their partner, most of us think it's smaller than whatever size we are! Realistically, the majority of us know when we've put on a few too many pounds, and have a clothes size we secretly hanker after or have something hanging in our wardrobe that we'd really like to fit into again one day. This plan is geared towards dropping a clothes size, but it can still work for you if you need to drop more than one size – provided you stay with it for long enough. And if you are significantly overweight – and more than half the UK population is now classified as such – you'll be doing yourself a huge favour by taking steps to lose those excess pounds.

Obesity is now recognized as a serious medical condition with many associated health risks, including heart disease, hypertension, diabetes, gallstones, osteo-arthritis of weight-bearing joints, sleep apnoea, reproductive disorders and some cancers. Professor Philip James, chairman of the Obesity Task Force, describes obesity as 'the biggest global health burden for the world'. And while the UK may lag behind the US in rates of obesity, we're gaining ground rapidly. In 1980, the average British man weighed 73.7kg; for a woman the average was 62.2kg. By 2000, those figures had increased to 81.6kg and 68.8kg respectively.

ASSESSING YOUR BODY MASS INDEX (BMI)

BMI is a simple way of assessing your body weight status. It's not foolproof, however, as it does not distinguish between fat and muscle. It's also not a good measure of progress as you get fitter, as increased muscle mass may actually make you heavier rather than lighter, although you will be substantially fitter and trimmer and slipping into a smaller clothes size.

Use the formula below to determine your BMI and then check this against the BMI categories to see whether you are already a healthy body weight or if you have a more significant amount of body fat to lose.

To obtain you BMI, measure your weight in kilograms and your height in metres and then divide your weight by your height squared: $W/H^2 = BMI$.

For example, if you weigh 63kg and are 1.70m tall, you multiply 1.7 by 1.7 to give you 2.89, then divide 63 by

2.89. This gives a BMI of 21.79, which, as you can see from the categories on page 8, would put you within the normal weight range. (If you want to make life easy, you can calculate your BMI automatically without having to do the maths at my website www.joannahallonline.com)

BMI CATEGORIES
Underweight = under 20
Normal weight = 20–24.9
Overweight = 25–29.9
Obese = 30+

WAIST CIRCUMFERENCE
Although BMI has been widely used since the 1980s to estimate body shape change and the risk of various obesity-related diseases, using the waist circumference measurement is simpler and has been shown to indicate obesity-related risks just as well as BMI. Developed by an expert panel on obesity and health risks, the waist circumference method of indicating health risk classifies a healthy waist circumference as being below 102cm/40in for men and 88cm/34in for women.

As well as being simple, the waist circumference measurement also gives a more accurate picture of an individual's body fat distribution. And since the Drop a Size for Life plan is concerned not solely with measuring weight on the scales but more with clothes size, girth measurements are the best way to monitor your progress as you follow this plan.

TAKING YOUR GIRTH MEASUREMENTS

The charts opposite shows the usual measurements that
are taken – if you wish you can use it to record you own
details when you begin the plan. The body fat measurement is not essential but it is helpful. Body fat can be
measured using skin fold calipers or, more conveniently,
using a body fat monitor – these are similar to bathroom
scales but they determine your percentage body fat, giving a truer idea of what is going on in your body.

For Women:	
Weight	
Body fat (if known)	
Chest	
Waist	
Navel	
Hips	
Thighs	

For Men:	
Weight	
Body fat (if known)	
Chest	
Waist with belly button contracted	
Waist with belly button relaxed	
Hips	
Thighs	

HOW TO MEASURE

Chest – measure with the tape flat across the nipple line

Waist – measure around the narrowest part of your midriff (for men, pull your tummy in for the first reading and let it go for the second)

Navel – measure around the midriff directly over the belly button

Hips – measure across the top of the buttock cheeks

Thighs – stand with feet together, measure 20cm/8in up from the top of your kneecap and take a circumference measurement of your thighs

SOME COMMON QUESTIONS

Can I drop a size just on my bottom half?

Unfortunately, you can't choose where the weight comes off. You might want to lose a size on your hips and gain one on your bust – no can do! The body loses fat from all over, not just from where you want it to. And the idea that you can 'burn' fat from specific areas – a concept known as spot reduction – is a myth. In fact, in one study, subjects performed a vast number of sit-ups over a few weeks and lost not a single gram of fat from their abdominal regions. However, an appropriate exercise program will help to firm up slack muscles and create a streamlined, balanced silhouette. This is one reason why exercise is such a crucial part of your DAS plan.

How long will it take to drop a size?
To drop a dress size, you need to lose at least 2.5cm/1in off your bust, 4cm/1.5in off your waist and 4cm/1.5in off your hips – that's a total of 10cm/4in. Men need to lose at least 2.5cm/1in from the waist and the same from the chest – a total of at least 5cm/2in. The amount of effort and time you are willing to put in will dictate how long it takes to drop a size (you can read more about this in section two) but don't be too impatient for results. Bear in mind the story of the tortoise and the hare. You can drop a size very quickly if you want to and if the time is right for you. All the volunteers who took part in the research for my previous book, *Drop a Size in Two Weeks Flat!*, dropped a whole size in just 14 days – and many of you have written to me to tell me you have too. However, it may not be the right time for you to drop a size in just two weeks and you may find it a lot more pleasurable and attainable if you take it a little more slowly. If you do it slowly you're also more likely to sustain the weight loss.

Will I always be able to stay at my new size?
In a word, no. As we age, physiological and metabolic processes slow down, often resulting in weight gain. This doesn't mean you'll inevitably gain weight, never to lose it. Life is continually changing and there will be times when it will be very hard to stay at your new size – you may even find that occasionally you gain a size. Conversely, there are times when the weight seems to just fall off without much

effort. Learning how to respond to your body's needs, both physically and mentally, will enable you to stay within a healthy weight range – and to return to your ideal size – throughout your life.

TAKE A REALITY CHECK

It is important to realize that how much weight you want to lose and how much is realistic in a given time frame may be two different things. Being realistic about what you can achieve is vital. How much time are you willing and able to put in? How many changes can you make at once? Weight loss isn't an all or nothing thing. Just because you won't fit into a size 10 by your next holiday, does that mean it's not worth doing at all? Think of approaching weight loss in terms of bite-size goals. What can you do right now? Now may not be the right time to go the whole hog, but that doesn't mean you can't do anything towards dropping a size.

Imagine you're relaxing with a group of friends, enjoying a bottle of wine and a bowl of tortilla chips while discussing the latest diet you'll start next Monday. The good intention is there, but it isn't a 'now' intention. Ask yourself what you can do now? Well for a start you can stop hogging the wine and eating most of the tortilla chips! You can ditch the sugar from your tea. At lunchtime, forgo the mayonnaise, butter and other added fats. Ask for skimmed milk in your cappuccino. Walk to school to pick up the kids instead of driving. It's the drip-drip effect — all these small things are positive steps towards your ultimate goal. Do what you can do now — and praise yourself for it.

HOW THE BOOK WORKS

Drop a Size for Life will help you master, develop and sustain the skills you need to lose weight and keep it off — and it will help you feel good about your body. I have written it in three simple-to-follow sections.

Section one is all about preparing to drop a size. It looks at how to get yourself mentally in the right place to lose weight. Many people want to drop a size, but in reality they are not in the right state of mind to do it. They may have a fear of failing, or have experienced great frustration with their weight loss efforts in the past, or they may simply be convinced that weight loss is some sort of losing–gaining, losing–gaining process. Such people resign themselves to starting a new diet every spring, rather than accepting that it is possible to lose weight and keep it off.

Finding the shape and size you are happy with is as much about your brain as your body. If you view your weight loss efforts as open warfare against your body, you'll be fighting against your best ally. Section one is about mastering six simple and easy-to-follow steps that form the foundation for you to drop a size for life. They centre around building your self-esteem, making friends with your body so you can work with it, strengthening your resolve and empowering you to be in control of your efforts. Achieve that and you'll not only look great but you'll feel good about yourself, too – and of course, you'll reap the rewards from the myriad health benefits of a nutritious diet and active lifestyle.

Section two is about dropping a size. This is the practical stuff about actually shedding those excess pounds. It includes eating and exercise plans that will provide you with a template to drop a size. As we go through the year our tastes change so I've provided summer and winter eating plans to help you keep that weight off all year round. When it comes to exercise, you'll find a 'workout wedge' that is suitable, whatever your available time and energy level. This section also includes ten vital strategies that underpin the plan – you can adopt these to whatever extent you feel necessary to make this work for you. And to help you stay in great shape, you'll find the drop a size for life foods and recipes offer you loads of ideas to keep you bursting with health and energy.

Section three is about staying at your new size throughout your life. As we age, our bodies naturally change shape, but how we manage the ageing process, our changing emotions, social lives and environment directly affects our bodies. Section three will take you through the changes associated with the different life stages, explaining what happens so that you don't feel that your body has suddenly turned against you. It will arm you with skills and strategies that are easy to slot into your life and that will help you navigate your way healthily and successfully through changing times. You'll also find helpful references to point you in the direction of relevant exercises and tips from sections one and two.

So, if you're ready, let's make a start and prepare to drop a size.

PREPARING TO DROP A SIZE

INTRODUCTION

Many people want to lose weight. What's the first step? I guess you'd expect to hear something about reducing calories and getting down the gym, however, my experience with the thousands of people I've helped over the years suggests that the first step should have nothing to do with diet or exercise – instead it should involve sorting out your state of mind. Getting in the right 'head space' – being mentally ready – is something you'll need to master for successful long-term weight management. Why? I see many clients with the keenness to achieve their weight loss goals, but they set off with false ideas – about how much they need to lose, how quickly it can be lost and how easy it will be. Attempting to achieve unrealistic goals means you are more likely to fail – either by not getting the result you wanted or by finding the plan too difficult to stick to and giving up. Either way, setting yourself up for failure in this way is bad for your self-esteem and confidence.

In contrast to those who are very keen, are the clients who have been through the weight loss mill so many times that despite saying, 'I really want to lose weight this time', at the back of their mind they are in fact saying 'here we go again – don't expect this will work but I'm desperate, so I'll give it a go'. In effect, they are setting themselves up to fail. The subconscious mind is a very subtle but persuasive thing and you only need to suggest failure for it to become a likely part of reality.

Many individuals report feelings of great self-esteem once they have lost weight. Why is that? Does being thinner make you a better person? Or is it more to do with the good feelings associated with achieving what you set out to do? Obviously losing weight doesn't make you a better person but whatever you think, I believe that building self-esteem initially is pivotal to successful weight loss. Self-esteem is not a **product** of weight loss but the **foundation** for it. After all, you have to believe you are worth the time, effort and work involved in achieving and then maintaining your goal size and weight.

Take your clothes off – go on, take them off right now. I'm absolutely serious! Go and take them off and stand in front of a full length mirror completely naked. Take a good look. Look at yourself from the front and then from the side and back. What do you see?

The chances are, what you see and the body you have are two completely different things. How you see yourself is described as your 'body image'. This isn't something fixed in concrete and it isn't necessarily grounded in reality. In fact, body image can be affected by all kinds of things. For example, in one interesting study, subjects who were made to consume a bowl of ice cream before having to choose a body silhouette most like their own opted for a larger outline than the women who ate nothing. It's as if those women felt they'd done something wrong by eating the ice cream and therefore judged themselves more negatively.

If you're anything like the average woman, you aren't at all happy with what you see in the mirror. A recent survey showed 95 per cent of women are unhappy with their body shape. What's more, we think that our inability to look as slim and fit as we want to is down to our own failures. Most disturbingly, 'failing' in one area of life (i.e. not having the 'perfect' body) has a knock-on effect on confidence and self-esteem in other areas of life. A negative body image is closely linked to poor self-esteem. The point here is that deciding to accept your body, right here, right now, how it is, is crucial to your success. Okay, so you might want to make some changes, but that doesn't mean you can't think positive about some aspects of yourself.

See if you can guess which of these percentages goes with which question.

Such widespread dissatisfaction with our bodies makes shocking reading, doesn't it? You are more than what you see in the mirror and to move beyond the crash diet–weight gain cycle, you need to accept yourself and value yourself enough to instigate some positive changes. Making an enemy of your body is a losing battle, as you will only be fighting yourself.

So, before we even begin to look at diet and exercise, we're going to work on getting you into the right mental space to drop a size for life. This section is literally about stripping things back to the bare bones and then building

60%   5%   90%   56%   0%   48%

1. A survey asked, 'would you change anything about your body if you had the chance?' What percentage said 'I'm happy as I am, thanks.'
2. What percentage of women overestimate their size?
3. What percentage of *normal weight* women report themselves overweight?
4. What percentage of British women are dieting at any one time?
5. What percentage of the female population can achieve the current media 'ideal' of thinness?
6. What percentage of survey respondents when asked, 'would you rather be thinner or smarter' said they'd prefer to drop pounds?

The answers are
1 (0%),
2 (90%),
3 (56%),
4 (60%),
5 (5%),
6 (48%)

back your self-esteem, layer by layer, in order to give you the appropriate foundation for dropping a size. And the great thing is, layering these simple skills and techniques will not only get you dropping a size, it will also have a knock-on effect in other aspects of your life, too.

HOW TO USE SECTION ONE

This section takes you through seven strategies that will help you understand the importance of engaging your mind – and not just your body – in your weight loss efforts. Each strategy builds upon the next, making each new one easier to understand and implement. Layer by layer the strategies build up, leading you towards your goal of creating the sort of mindset needed to drop a size for life.

Because each strategy builds the foundation for the next, you will need to go through each one methodically, and feel happy with it, before you can successfully tackle the next. You may find some of the steps easier to master than others, but do not be tempted to skip any – each one is an important aspect of your journey to drop a size and keep it off.

This section isn't something you'll go through once and then forget about. As you go through life there will be times when your weight fluctuates – when events in your life may knock your confidence, affecting your mindset – and you need to get back on track. At such

STEP ONE: TRAIN YOUR BRAIN

The point of training your brain is to increase mind-body synergy – which basically means that your brain and body should be singing from the same hymn sheet! If you are trying to force your body to do something without your brain's support, you are much more likely to fail.

We are all aware that in order to lose weight we need to make some big changes to our energy intake and expenditure. But for us to see a change in our bodies and to actually drop that size we need to work on the relationship between brain and body. For our bodies to lose weight, yes, we have to eat less and exercise more, but for the mind's eye image in the mirror to change, we need to get our brain on the winning side, too.

The mind is a crucial factor in weight loss success because what we think about ourselves can give significant momentum to our efforts and hence directly affect the result of those efforts. If your brain is not on the same wavelength as your body then your weight loss efforts will flounder. I have seen it time and time again with my clients – however, once they have mastered these seven simple steps they achieve greater success and it lasts longer too!

Not getting your mind sorted out before you embark on your weight loss plan is a bit like setting off on holiday without any preparation – you can't wait to get there and you're so excited about arriving quickly you don't bother to check the oil, water and petrol gauge before you set off and end up breaking down. You might have been raring to go, but the car wasn't and the upshot is you end up stuck on the hard shoulder for 2 hours waiting to be rescued. If you'd taken a little time to ensure the car was as ready for the journey as you were, you'd be well on your way. Instead, the journey that you were so excited about has become tediously long, disappointing and irritating. Of course, in reality, few of us would set out on a long and important journey without checking the basics, yet many of us embark on our weight loss journey without seeing to the fundamentals first!

The action points for step one are all about getting your brain to register what you are feeling within your body, thus forging a closer link between mind and body.

ACTION POINT 1: TIME YOURSELF

WHAT YOU NEED TO DO

Time how long it takes you to eat your meals. Time each meal separately – your breakfast, lunch, dinner and snacks. You may find you wolf down your breakfast and lunch, but have a more leisurely dinner. Alternatively, dinner may be a hurried affair as you try to eat your main meal while simultaneously feeding the kids, or you simply race through it so you can collapse on the sofa and have a rest.

Once you have recorded your times, try to give yourself longer to complete each meal. Start off by aiming to increase the amount of time it takes to eat each meal by 50 per cent. Try to do this for each meal for one whole week. In the following week, try to add a further 50 per cent of time to complete each meal.

THE LOGIC

It takes 20 minutes for the stretch receptors in your stomach lining to send a message to the brain registering there is any food inside. As a result, when you are full there is a gap before the brain actually receives a message to that effect – by that time you may well have eaten more calories than you actually need.

Eating too quickly is itself unwise. It can cause digestive problems and has been acknowledged as a factor in irritable bowel syndrome. In reality, your life may not allow you to devote more time to all your meals, but even the process of doing it sometimes will make you more aware not just of what you are eating, but how much you are eating. Eating will become more of a conscious process rather than an unconscious motion that happens as life rushes on around you.

ACTION POINT 2: EAT UNTIL YOU ARE
80 PER CENT FULL

WHAT YOU NEED TO DO

You know what 100 per cent full feels like, so back off before you reach that point. At first, eating until you're about 80 per cent full may feel an alien thing to do – perhaps you were always told to finish everything on your plate as a child, or your body just really likes that feeling of being very full – but persevere with this, it has multiple benefits.

THE LOGIC

Your schedule may not allow you to always take as much time as you would like over each meal or snack, so learning to eat until you are 80 per cent full is a back-up plan that works hand-in-hand with taking more time over your food. This allows your brain to become aware of the food entering your body, which stops you from over-eating and actually energizes you more. Eating too much food decreases your immediate energy levels, as your body has to work harder through a process called the 'thermic effect of feeding' to digest your food. This can leave you devoid of energy and feeling as if you need to reach for that chocolate bar for an instant energy fix. In addition, you should start to feel empowered as you feel more in control of your food volume. Saying no can be very powerful.

ACTION POINT 3: EAT WITHOUT DISTRACTIONS

WHAT YOU NEED TO DO

Try to eat your meals without any distractions. In your lunch break, stop trying to finish off a report as you munch at a sandwich; at breakfast, avoid grabbing mouthfuls of toast in between applying your mascara and ironing your blouse for work. Okay, okay, I hear you say – where am I going to find the time to do this? Well, I do understand that you may not be able to do it for *all* your meals for the *whole* week, but do try to do it at least once for each meal during the course of your first week. Try to focus entirely on the food on your plate – look at the colours before you start to eat, feel the texture of the food in your mouth and chew your food completely before you swallow.

THE LOGIC

Today's fast-paced lifestyles mean that eating meals gets put on the 'to do' list as we multi-task with other aspects of our busy day. However, eating should not be a task – it should be an enjoyable experience that you share with friends or take time over. Sadly, it has become so rushed that we no longer seem to appreciate what we are eating or the actual sensual pleasure eating can give us. Eating can be sexy! Taking the time to really concentrate on and relish your food will heighten your awareness and sensuality of food. Focus on both the amount you are eating and the way it feels as it enters your body.

ACTION POINT 4: BELT UP!

WHAT YOU NEED TO DO

Stop wearing elasticated waistbands. Replace them with fitted waistbands or belts. Do this straightaway, not tomorrow, not next week, but straightaway. You need a reference point that tells you how much space your body takes up and this will help your brain to become aware of this.

THE LOGIC

Elasticated waistbands lull you into a false sense of security. They encourage your abdominal muscles to become lazy, as there is no reference point for your tummy muscles to press against. Although it sounds rather insignificant, changing to inflexible waistbands is a very effective act. Firstly, by changing to a rigid belt you are able to mark your progress on your belt notches. Secondly, the act of changing to a rigid belt is a positive step towards getting to know your body better.

If your clothes only have elasticated waistbands, tie a thick piece of ribbon around your midriff under your clothes. Fix it firmly so you can feel it around your waist without it digging into you – this will give you a reference point of where your body ends and the belt begins. If you are a man, your task is to stop lowering your waistband so it lies under your beer belly. This only further lulls you into a false sense of security that your belly really isn't that big. You don't have to wear your trousers under your ribcage but you do need to start accepting the 'real waist' situation. And, as a bonus, doing this will improve your posture.

THE BOTTOM LINE

Like any relationship worth sustaining, the brain-body link needs attention and care in order to remain strong. Don't become lazy in maintaining mind-body awareness. Once you have fostered a closer relationship between your brain and body, you are ready for step two.

Case Study: Rebecca's Story

'Although I was desperate to lose weight, all the diets I had read about involved cutting out all the foods that I enjoyed the most: chocolate, biscuits, pies, chips, lasagne, cheese, mayonnaise, quiche etc. To have to consider giving them all up was just too daunting. Then I read the Drop a Size plan. First of all I increased my water intake – that alone gave me energy. I didn't feel so groggy all the time and was able to think more clearly. Within a couple of weeks my body began to ask for water – it had become automatic. I made up my mind that, while I would make healthier choices, if I needed a chocolate fix I would have one, but a small one. By Christmas I was close to being ready to start dieting. January 2nd was 'D' Day – Diet Day. But I didn't go all out. I wanted to be kind to myself and ease myself into the process in a way considerate to my needs. I knew myself, and my limitations, and I wanted to succeed, so I made it challenging but not scary.

For the first couple of weeks of following the Carb Curfew I went to bed in the evening with a light feeling in my stomach that was alien to me. Before, my usual evening meal was meat, sometimes vegetables (not always) and potatoes or rice or pasta. I was so accustomed to feeling heavy, lethargic and sometimes bloated that I thought it was normal. The extra energy I had in the evenings gave me the motivation to exercise. It was all beginning to snowball and I was feeling really good. Only when I began to feel some of my clothes a little looser did I venture on to the scales. I had lost 4lbs. It was the incentive I needed to carry on.'

STEP TWO: BEFRIEND
THE MIRROR

As we cast a critical eye over our bodies in the mirror, many of us focus on one particular body part. When you stripped off and assessed yourself, did you find yourself honing straight in on your much-hated hips or tummy? If so, you probably felt pretty negative about yourself by the time you turned away from the mirror. That's why it's important to look beyond the mirror and acknowledge that your reflection is not all you are. Think about all the things your body can do, the pleasure it can provide, the miracles it has performed, the strength, endurance and power it has. Think how great it feels when you get massaged, or when you stretch after waking up or after a workout; how good it feels to slip into a hot bath, eat something delicious or dance. All these things are about your body and the way it feels, the way it performs, the way it can be challenged. Your body is so much more than that reflection you are so critical of.

Imagine seeing yourself through the eyes of one of your friends. How would you describe your body if you were to look at it as an outsider? Write that description down now, being as honest and accurate as you can be. The chances are if you're looking at yourself through someone else's eyes you'll be a lot kinder, so use these more realistic judgements when you're casting a critical eye over yourself and determining your goals and objectives. The reality is that everyone has good and bad points. Having a big bum, a beer belly or flabby upper arms doesn't make you a bad person, a failure, or in any way a lesser being than the supermodels that pout at us from the pages of countless glossy magazines.

ACTION POINT 1: ACKNOWLEDGE THE POSITIVE

WHAT YOU NEED TO DO

Look at your reflection in the mirror and find one physical thing about yourself you like. It can be anything from the shape of your little toe, to the way your nose wrinkles when you smile, or the shape of your ankles. Whatever it is, find one thing and tell yourself out loud why you like it.

THE LOGIC

Acknowledging something you like about your body shifts the emphasis away from the bits you don't like. By doing this you start to see your body as a whole rather than as a collection of isolated bits. This will help you feel more positive about your body and, because you feel better about it, you will use it in a more positive way.

ACTION POINT 2: BUILD UP YOUR GOOD POINTS

WHAT YOU NEED TO DO

As the days pass, find another aspect of your body you like and say it out loud, along with the bits you liked from previous days. For example, if on day one you said 'I like my little toe', then on day two repeat this out loud together with the next body bit that you like. Continue to add a new 'like' each day until you are repeating a lengthy list of aspects of your body that you like.

THE LOGIC

Reinforcement is a powerful tool in helping you believe in something.

ACTION POINT 3: MAKE IT YOURS!

WHAT YOU NEED TO DO

Think about precisely why you like each body bit and repeat these reasons out loud as you look in the mirror.

THE LOGIC

Personalizing why you like these good bits helps you develop a closer relationship with your body and encourages you to like your body for reasons beyond conventional beauty. This will help you challenge your thought process on what makes someone beautiful or acceptable. Quirkiness can actually be to your benefit, so learn to embrace all the parts of your body so you can make friends with what you see in the mirror instead of criticizing it.

ACTION POINT 4: PAY YOURSELF A GENUINE COMPLIMENT

WHAT YOU NEED TO DO

I want you to pay yourself a genuine compliment each morning as you look in the mirror. Choose a different compliment each day – it can relate to you physically or be about something you have accomplished in your life. Whatever it is, you need to say it out loud as you look at yourself in the mirror.

THE LOGIC

Seeing your reflection is about facing up to who you are physically, but it is also about acknowledging that there are many facets to the person you see in the mirror. Accepting and praising yourself for all your qualities helps you to accept yourself physically, mentally and spiritually. Being content with yourself is not just about whether you are beautiful, but about whether you pulled off a great project at work, hosted a fab dinner party, dried your hair really nicely, were patient with the kids this morning or didn't shout at your boyfriend for forgetting to put the rubbish out.

ACTION POINT 5: PLAY TO WIN

WHAT YOU NEED TO DO

Acknowledge the great things you have achieved in your life. Take credit for your accomplishments and don't belittle your achievements by dismissing your work as merely 'okay' or 'not bad' – use bold, positive words that truly reflect your accomplishments. Shout it out!

THE LOGIC

Too many of us down play our triumphs – particularly professional ones – so others feel more secure. At school we are taught to be modest – a 'good girl' was one who promoted the people around her and not herself. This modesty can actually undermine and sabotage confidence, because as we progress through our lives, fewer and fewer of us receive compliments or feedback on our performance. If you lack the ability to acknowledge and even shout about your own accomplishments, they can start to go unnoticed by the most important person – YOU. If you don't value what you do, it's a cue for others to do the same.

THE BOTTOM LINE

Making friends with the mirror is a two-pronged strategy. It's about accepting what you see and also about acknowledging that being you isn't simply about squeezing into a particular size. The mirror can never reflect the myriad aspects and depths of your personality and being. Once you have accepted this, you are ready to move on to step three.

Case Study: Diane's Success

'When I met Joanna Hall in November 2002 at the *This Morning* studio, I had reached an end point. I was unhappy with my weight – I wanted to lose at least 2 stone but the thought of dieting was intimidating. For a lot of my adult life I had been plagued by depression and one of my comforts was to eat. I was ashamed of myself and that turned the whole situation into a vicious circle. If you asked me what was the most important factor in my successful weight loss, I would have to say a positive mind. I needed encouragement, but more than that I needed to be able to believe in myself. Joanna suggesting coming at it from a different angle and helped me to build my self-esteem and confidence, showing me how important it is to like, even love, myself. She gave me the building blocks to change my mindset to one that was able to take on the challenge of losing weight.'

STEP THREE: THINK, SAY AND DO AS ONE

This step is about making the relationship you've now established between your brain and body work. When you do something it involves a three-stage process: you THINK about it, you SAY you're going to do it and then you take the necessary action – you DO it. So, for example, with weight loss, you think about your dissatisfaction with your current size and how you would like to change it, you talk about introducing diet and exercise into your life and then you take the appropriate steps to help you reach your weight loss goals. Or do you? It seems obvious enough that all these three things need to be going in the same direction, but do we actually do it?

Take Susan's story: Susan thought she had great big wobbly bits that stuck out from the sides of her thighs like saddlebags. In fact, her thighs only measured 90cm/36in but, to her, they were very large. She wanted to lose weight, so she gave herself a talking to and told her friends – when they were out at the cinema having ice cream – that she would be starting her campaign in earnest the next day. She had bought the latest diet sensation – it came with a government health warning, but what the heck! Oh, and she was going to get up and run every morning, and again when she came home from work. Yet despite all this positive talk, Susan felt deep down that she would still have her saddlebags. What Susan *thought*, *said* and *did* were not all going in the same direction.

She said she was going to take action and she did do what she said she would, but since she believed that she would fail, and still have her saddlebags at the end of it, her thoughts were going in a different direction to her words and actions. After a time, this would inevitably sabotage her efforts.

When what you do, or what you say you will do, is based on negative thoughts about yourself – a limiting belief – this negativity can only grow. It's like feeding a fire. When you want to light a fire you get your kindling, some dry newspaper, wood and some firelighters and as the fire starts to burn you apply a little more air to fuel it. The more air you provide at the base, the fiercer the fire grows. Your thoughts are the same – they fuel the fire of your actions. Therefore if your fundamental belief is that you are going to fail, then you are more likely to – and of course each time you do, it will only serve to fuel your negativity and make it stronger, which makes losing weight harder each time you try.

Think about where you were five years ago and imagine a straight line from there to here, the present moment.

Now extend that line into the future – by continuing to do as you do now, you'll be where in five years time? If that place isn't where you want to be, you need to change direction by addressing your thinking, saying and doing right now.

ACTION POINT 1: ESTABLISH THE PAY-OFF

WHAT YOU NEED TO DO

Make a list of at least five ways you think you will benefit by dropping a size and being more physically active. Be specific about what the benefit will be to you and how it will personally affect you. For example, having more energy is a common benefit, but to empower this statement and make it personal to you, you may need to write something like, 'When I drop a size, I will have the energy to enjoy more intimacy with my partner.'

THE LOGIC

Writing things down makes you embrace your thoughts and the visual images this creates can reinforce what you think. Personalizing your benefit also allows you to see how your actions will directly affect you. Keeping these benefits personal rather than general makes them more appropriate to you and hence they become more powerful motivators. So stop being general and be more specific!

ACTION POINT 2: LIST YOUR SUCCESSES

WHAT YOU NEED TO DO
Make a list of all the things you have previously thought
you would like to do in your life and have since accomplished. This list can cover small things such as cooking
your first three-course meal or changing your own flat
tyre. As long as you saw it as a challenge and you succeeded, it counts.

THE LOGIC
The action of recalling events or situations in which you
have overcome a challenge helps reassure you that you
have the potential to translate your thinking and saying
into a successful action.

ACTION POINT 3: FIND YOUR MANTRA

WHAT YOU NEED TO DO
This is about making belief part of your thoughts. Think
of five positive affirmations for yourself. You need to be
able to really believe in them – and they must be positively stated. Here is one of my client's mantras: 'I am going
to do this for me. Steve Redgrave is my age and if he, as a
man of my age, can take responsibility for his health then
I can take responsibility for mine.'

THE LOGIC

Mantras can provide the positive momentum to get you where you need to be. They help strengthen your self-belief and build a strong foundation for your actions.

ACTION POINT 4: COMMIT TO PAPER

WHAT YOU NEED TO DO

Write your mantras down and place them in your under-wear drawer, in your office drawer, on the mirror that you look at first thing in the morning, on a scrap of paper in your purse – anywhere that will reinforce your thought line.

THE LOGIC

Reinforcement works, even at a subconscious level.

ACTION POINT 5: TRACE YOUR ACTIONS

WHAT YOU NEED TO DO

Draw a table with three columns. At the top of each column write what you have thought, said and did with regard to diet and weight loss in the past, then write down your intentions this time round (you may find it helpful to revise this once you've read section two). On page 44 is an example of thinking, saying and doing not going in the same direction, followed by an example of when they do go in the same direction.

Think	Say	Do
It's going to be so difficult to shift this post-baby weight	I'm going to do 100 sit-ups every morning and eat one meal a day	Attempt the sit-ups and calorie deprivation regime for 3 days and end up knackered with a cold

Think	Say	Do
I will shift this post-baby weight, slowly but surely	I'm going to walk for 15 minutes every day with the buggy, fit in toning exercises when baby Grace is asleep and make a job lot of healthy soups and stews that I can freeze	Buy a good home exercise video with short, effective routines. Find a support network, such as a text messaging service to your mobile phone, to stay on track. Begin walking and compromise on the healthy eating by making a batch of soup and buying some low-fat ready-meals

THE LOGIC

Committing your thoughts, aims and actions to paper allows you to see whether they are all heading the right way. Your past experience may also offer some clues as to pitfalls to avoid. If your thoughts are undermining your aims and actions, go back to your mantras, ensure they are positively stated and that you are saying and seeing them every day.

THE BOTTOM LINE

Ensuring that what you think, say and do are all heading in the same direction means your mind and body are primed for positive action. Achieve this and you are ready for step four.

Case study: Maxine's Success

'Joanna's approach is so easy to implement – for us, it's become a way of life. We've made small changes and haven't missed the carbs in the evening. Aside from the practicalities, it's worked because it has helped me look at myself differently. In the past I always felt low when losing weight, but this time I'm so much more positive.

Before I felt a nobody, a nothing – now I feel like somebody and worth something. I used to hate myself, but Joanna has helped me build my self-esteem so that I now actually like myself. I may still beat myself up a bit if I have a "bad day" but Joanna has taught me to put this in proportion and not let one blip ruin everything or make me feel like a failure. Now I feel nice in some of my clothes – and I've never felt like that! My mantra was "I'm going to like what I see – this is me" now it's "I like what I see – this is me"! And Joanna's tip about making my mantra my welcome note on my mobile is great – now it's always there for me to see!

My husband has even followed the plan and he's a butcher! He's gone from 18 stone 2 pounds to 16 stone – a weight he never expected to achieve, and he's managed to stay at it too.'

Maxine lost 30lbs and dropped from a size 24 to 16–18.

STEP FOUR: MAKE FRIENDS
WITH THE ENEMY

This strategy is about embracing whatever issue has stopped you from successfully losing weight in the past. Body weight can be closely linked to emotional issues, therefore both gain and loss can be directly affected by and associated with events in our lives. Traumatic or highly significant events and turning points can trigger an unhealthy relationship with our bodies, and with food and dieting, all of which can culminate in a decreased level of self-worth and self-esteem.

The step four action points are about facing up to your fears and enemies.

ACTION POINT 1: REVISIT PAST ACTS OF
BRAVERY AND FEARLESSNESS

WHAT YOU NEED TO DO
If you are feeling demoralized or unable to face a situation for fear of rejection or failure, then recounting previous acts of bravery can help you see that you are a brave person and that you can face up to difficulties. To trigger

these memories sketch out a time line spanning from
kindergarten to adult life. Try to jot down ten courageous
acts. If you cannot remember, ask a friend or older mem-
ber of the family. Make a list of events you have feared in
your life and beside them write down the outcome of the
event or situation.

THE LOGIC

Revisiting the past and citing even the smallest of brave
acts can remind you of your bravery. As we get older our
brain often forgets these small acts and instead we tend to
focus on what we feel we have not been able to address and
overcome. Even the most timid of people will have had
fearless moments – the trick is to remind yourself.

ACTION POINT 2: SAY YOUR MANTRA

WHAT YOU NEED TO DO

Once you have your bravery time line, you can use it as a
springboard to a powerful mantra such as 'I was brave once,
I can be brave again'. Repeat your mantra every morning
and also write it down and place it in an area where your
confidence is most challenged. If this is at work, for example, keep it in the top drawer of your desk. Alternatively, you
could make it your welcome message when you switch on
your mobile phone. Wherever you choose, make sure it is
somewhere where you will see it regularly – the more you
see it, the more powerful its effect on you.

THE LOGIC

Mantras are powerful sayings but they can only be put to good effect if you use them wisely and allow them to reinforce your feelings when needed.

ACTION POINT 3: STEP INTO THE TARDIS

WHAT YOU NEED TO DO

Make a list of past situations or events that you were fearful of or worried about. Next, write down whether you feel you dealt with that situation or event successfully or not. Now write down how you dealt with the situation and, finally, note how you think you could have improved the outcome by using a different approach or strategy.

THE LOGIC

Addressing situations that have caused you hurt or problems in the past, and how you have dealt with them, allows you to accept that your attitude to weight management needs to involve a series of strategies and approaches to achieve the outcome you want. It also enables you to see how you have been able to work through various other situations in your life, and that the outcome has not always been immediate.

ACTION POINT 4: THINK CHALLENGE, NOT PROBLEM

WHAT YOU NEED TO DO

This relates to whether you see your glass as half full or half empty. Decide right now that it is half full. This outlook will motivate you and provide you with more energy to address the issue.

THE LOGIC

How you view a situation can have a significant impact on how you feel about it and how you deal with it, so stop looking at the difficulties life throws at you as problems and instead see them as challenges that present new ways for you to look at your life and learn about yourself and others.

ACTION POINT 5: STOP WORRYING WHAT OTHERS THINK

WHAT YOU NEED TO DO

Observe any young child and you will see them playing silly games, or dancing as if they're the latest pop sensation, with no regard to how silly they look. When was the last time you did something silly or put yourself in an unfamiliar situation without worrying about what others thought, or how ridiculous you may look? Fear of embarrassment can limit your experience of life. So take up belly dancing, audition for a part in a local theatre group or sign up for that evening class you have been thinking about for months. Go out power walking, or join the gym – and remember, the only person who is really focused on you is YOU.

THE LOGIC

Not caring what others think is a liberating experience. It opens you to new experiences, building your confidence and self-esteem, and shows you that falling flat on your face once in a while isn't the end of the world. You'll be surprised how little attention others really give to all the small things you worry about.

ACTION POINT 6: DARE TO DO WHAT YOU FEAR

WHAT YOU NEED TO DO

As adults, many of us tend to protect ourselves emotion-ally and physically. Yet if you allow your fears to spin out to their worst-case conclusions, you'll find that the poten-tial consequences are usually manageable. What is the worst thing that can happen? Thinking it through can eliminate fear and provide you with the courage to move forward. Make a list of small things that would take you out of your comfort zone and try to do one a month for the next six months. Start with really tiny things, then make each one a little tougher.

THE LOGIC

When you are young you think you can do anything and not get hurt, but as we get older our limitations become instilled. Once you realize you are breakable and could end up in a plaster cast – or with a broken heart – it can dissuade you from trying anything more daring or stepping outside your comfort zone. Facing fears head-on will build your confidence and help you embrace change and challenges with improved confidence and vigour.

ACTION POINT 7: BE AN EARLY BIRD

WHAT YOU NEED TO DO

Each day, aim to do the things you least want to do, but have to do that day, first. It's like a child who leaves their favourite food on the plate till last and then eats it. If you tackle things in this way, you won't need to nag yourself all day about not getting it done – instead you will be able to deal with it and your positive action will empower you through the other activities in your day.

THE LOGIC

As well as avoiding the negative situation of having something unpleasant looming all day long, research shows that we are better able to deal with challenging situations in the morning, as levels of the stress hormones cortisol and adrenaline are naturally higher at this time. So make the most of your biochemicals!

THE BOTTOM LINE

Acknowledge that sadness, fear and other negative emotions can help you learn and heal, as well as helping you to celebrate and get the most out of life. Once you have made friends with the enemy you are ready for step five.

Case Study: Nikki's Story

Nikki, who was a victim of physical abuse, put weight on as a protective mechanism, a way of hiding behind the pain. She felt that if she made herself larger then the pain would be less and if she made herself, in her eyes, less attractive, then the physical abuse would stop. Repeatedly Nikki used this strategy whenever she hit difficult times in her life – when she was unhappy in her job, in her other personal relationships, had a row with her family or felt depressed from a family bereavement. Only when Nikki began to acknowledge what had happened to her, could she begin to see that overeating was her way of dealing with it. In this way she began the process of understanding her feelings and building her self-esteem. By mastering this step, Nikki went on to lose 18 pounds and drop 3 dress sizes.

Case Study: Elaine's Story

Elaine had always been slim and sporty as a teenager and in the early stages of her relationship with Chris. When Chris was asked to move to a new town with his job, he assumed Elaine would go with him and threatened to end the relationship if she didn't. As a result, Elaine gave up her own job and moved. However, with no social circle of her own and no work, her confidence suffered and she soon began taking comfort in food. Having gained nearly 13kg/2 stone, she found Chris was constantly criticizing her appearance and their sex life became non-existent. To make matters worse, he hardly included her in his own social life. It wasn't until Elaine had to move back to her home town to look after her mother, who was ill, that she was able to look at the situation calmly and see that her eating was a way of hiding her fear that without Chris she was nothing. She began exercising again and joined a slimming club and is now restarting her life without Chris.

STEP FIVE: ESTABLISHING THE HERE AND NOW

There are two phases to this strategy: the first is establishing where you are and the second is doing a reality check.

You may have an event in the not too distant future that you want to lose weight for – perhaps it's a wedding or a beach holiday. You know what you want to achieve – where you want to get to – but, before you embark on any plan, you need to establish where you are right here, right now. Losing weight and keeping it off is about what you do in the future, but it is also what you can do at this very moment, right here, right now. Yes, long-term weight loss is about what you carry on doing, but many people live in a twilight zone of not appreciating what they can do now, in this *actual* moment, to improve their health, feel better about themselves and lose weight.

Focusing too much on the future causes unhappiness because it prevents us from enjoying the moment. The brain is whirling ahead, thinking about dinner that night or worrying about little Johnny's report at the parents' evening next week, or your appraisal with your boss at the end of the month. All this chatter going on in the brain can dull your experience and enjoyment of what is happening now. It builds to create a toxic thought process that blocks your enjoyment of the moment and masks your perception of what you could do right now to help you towards your goal.

Once you have mastered the here and now skill, dropping a size becomes a sequence of 'now' moments that act as building blocks to successful long-term weight loss. When you have accepted that life is a series of 'nows', all joined up, you need to do a reality check and think about what is possible right now in terms of your weight loss efforts. Losing weight and keeping it off is a journey. It may be that life is very hectic for you at the current time – perhaps you're starting a new job and you've got the builders in – and you're not in the right 'space' to lose weight with as much effort or as fast as you would like. That's all right – don't beat yourself up about it. While I don't want to give you an excuse to put off what you can do today until tomorrow, there are many situations that can make it difficult to drop that size as quickly as you would like. That's just life – you need to do what you can when you can. In fact, perhaps you need to simply accept that staying the same size, rather than gaining a size, is a more realistic interim goal.

If you're trying to lose weight in a specific time frame and your life is not in the right space to allow you to achieve it, you need to change the time span you set yourself to lose that size.

Step five action aims are about learning to live in the NOW.

ACTION POINT 1: FORGIVE YOURSELF

WHAT YOU NEED TO DO

Start right now by saying sorry to yourself. Say sorry for the way you have given yourself a hard time over an issue in your life, no matter how big or small. For example, perhaps you feel that your lack of time and effort led to the breakdown of your relationship or you feel bad that you got caught up at work and were late picking up your child. Stop beating yourself up over it – acknowledge why it happened and forgive yourself for it. Then move forward.

THE LOGIC

Criticizing and blaming yourself is like telling your subconscious mind that you are a bad human being – and it will believe you. Everyone screws up sometimes, but the important thing is to acknowledge the error or mishap and move on. The scary fact is that giving yourself a hard time and getting stressed over it can, in the long term, make you fat. Negative emotions, such as depression, guilt and cynicism, are associated with higher levels of abdominal fat according to a study from Pennsylvania State University. Harbouring negative feelings won't help you achieve anything, but building and nurturing your self-esteem will.

Feeling guilty or angry with yourself about small things or day-to-day events is one thing, but if your whole life is dominated by negative emotions related to something that has taken place in your life, you may need the help of a counsellor or therapist in addressing these issues. However, remember one thing; whatever you did then, and whatever you do now, you have a responsibility to yourself to do the best you can – with the resources available to you – to boost your self-worth.

ACTION POINT 2: EMBRACE REALITY

WHAT YOU NEED TO DO

This is about doing a reality check to see where you are in your life right now. Perhaps you want to drop a size in two weeks, but since you have a major report to write for work, your tax return to do, and oh – you forgot – the in-laws are coming to stay …. it really isn't a realistic option. However, dropping a size over the next three months and taking what action you can right NOW, is possible. So assess where you are – is it the right time to go all-out, or is your current lifestyle more conducive to a longer-term approach? Whatever is right for you, you will find the appropriate strategies to help you in section two.

THE LOGIC

One of the most prevalent weight loss blunders that people make is embarking on a weight loss plan when the time simply isn't right. By doing this, they set themselves up for failure and, as a result of failing, reinforce any deep-seated feelings that they aren't capable of losing weight. However, this doesn't mean I'm giving people carte blanche to succumb to a tray of chocolate éclairs because the time isn't right to lose weight! At difficult times you need to set yourself small, realistic goals that you can achieve in the here and now. The next action point will tell you how.

ACTION POINT 3: OPEN YOUR DIARY

WHAT YOU NEED TO DO

Look at your diary and write down what you can physically do today that will help you to drop that size. Perhaps it is getting that 10-minute walk in before you eat your lunch, or meeting your friend to look around the shops rather than sitting in the coffee shop eating chocolate cakes. Plan a positive action for every day of the week – even if it's simply doing squats while the kettle boils or drinking a glass of water for each cup of coffee you drink.

THE LOGIC

Opening your diary makes you face your day, helping you to plan ahead and make a written commitment to yourself.

It also demonstrates that even though you aren't on a full-on diet and exercise program, you are still taking positive steps towards improving your health and, ultimately, dropping a size.

ACTION POINT 4: PRESS THE PAUSE BUTTON

WHAT YOU NEED TO DO

When did you last take five minutes just for you and did nothing, absolutely nothing – and that includes writing of lists (I apologize, as I have asked you to write a few so far in this book) or planning. When was the last time you actually let your brain be still? Start by finding three times a week (every day would be fab – but I am realistic) just for you. This can be difficult, but if you really cannot find five minutes in your existing day then I encourage you to set your alarm early to have this sacred time. Yes, your sleep is important but so is your sanity!

THE LOGIC

Finding space in your day to simply stop and 'be' rather than 'do' may seem difficult, or even a waste of valuable time, but pressing the pause button can actually be energizing and help you use your time more effectively later on.

Case study: Anita's Story

'It took me a while to get my head around the idea of following a specific weight loss program as I had just come out of feeding my second child – after 18 months of not being allowed to eat/drink my favourite things, I was suddenly voluntarily depriving myself! But since I'd gained 4½ stone since my second pregnancy, I wanted to go slow but remain in for the long-term – rather than do an incredible quick fix, rest on my laurels and then slip back again. My current weight/body fat shows that this approach has been a great success – it has really worked for me. It's been a fantastic kickstart to better all-round health and energy levels.'

THE BOTTOM LINE

Many of us spend our lives waiting for the perfect moment to lose weight, join the gym, embark on a difficult project ... However, that time may never come so do what you can, now! It might not be what you'd like to be able to do, but it's infinitely better than doing nothing because it empowers you – it means you are taking control and moving closer towards your goal. Once you've learned to work with the here and now, you are ready for step six.

STEP SIX: GET ON THAT PEDESTAL

This strategy is about raising yourself up your priority list. Where do you figure on your list of priorities? Ask yourself the following series of questions and write the answers down. Who is the most important person in your life? After that, who is the next most important person in your life? Ask yourself this question seven times. Next, take a piece of paper and play hangman, adding a new piece to the gallows for each name that appears on your list. If you get to six or seven before you reach your name, you're done for! Why? Because if you are that low down on your priority list, then your weight loss attempts will fail – they'll fail because your needs are not important enough for you to give them the time and energy they require. Quite simply, you do not value yourself enough.

Now ask yourself who is responsible for keeping all those other important people or things going and working in your life – chances are it's *you*. Let's get one thing straight: if you feel low about yourself, your health suffers through a lack of quality sleep and too little physical activity and this in turn makes sensible eating and other lifestyle choices harder. However, it's not only you who suffers as a result of this, but your family and anyone else you've put above you on your priority list.

Case Study: Katie and the hangman

Katie took part in one of my group weight management courses. A mother of three, she was frustrated about not being able to lose the weight she had gained since having Jessie, Amy and Matthew. She wanted to lose the weight, but kept getting sidetracked by all the other demands on her attention. She felt exasperated and upset that although she was doing so much for her family, she was also silently begrudging them for it. Playing the hangman game showed Katie how she needed to raise herself up the priority list. This is the list Katie came up with:

Michael my husband
Amy – as she was born with a heart condition
Matthew and Jessie
Mum
Sister
In-laws
Best friend Sue
Me

Seeing a visual depiction of the situation helped Katie put things into perspective. She knew she would never be number one – that was not her nature – but she knew by carving out a little time for herself and building even a small pedestal for herself would help with her weight loss efforts and help her feel less exasperated with the rest of the family.

TAKING AND MAKING TIME

Many people complain that they do not have enough time to eat healthily, take regular exercise and manage stress, but the issue is not about *making* time it is about *taking* time. Taking time is only possible when you feel you are worthy of it. Being happy to take time involves you raising yourself a few rungs up the ladder. Even if you are not at the top of the list, getting higher is important.

Step five action aims are about getting you to put yourself on a pedestal.

ACTION POINT 1: REPEAT AFTER ME – TAKING TIME FOR ME IS A WIN-WIN STRATEGY FOR EVERYONE

WHAT YOU NEED TO DO

Stop thinking that taking time out for you is selfish. Self-neglect is one of the most common issues I see in the women I work with – they are successful, run a happy home, excel at work, the fridge is full and family is always fed, but they end up going to bed way after everyone else, toss and turn worrying about all the things they need to do and end up even more tired the following day. Taking time out for you does not mean you are neglecting others – see it as looking after the main cog in the wheel of your family.

THE LOGIC
Saying this mantra will act as a powerful springboard to help you *want* to make self-care part of your schedule. It will help you make time for it, as opposed to simply finding time for it. Taking time out can help you, your family and others realize the pivotal role you play.

ACTION POINT 2: REBEL!

WHAT YOU NEED TO DO
Go on, do it – be a rebel. Stop loading yourself with pressure to be perfect. Go against the grain, step out of line, be edgy, say something shocking – anything that makes you feel you are being non-conformist and takes you out of the role others see you in.

THE LOGIC
Challenging others to view you in a slightly different light can help you look at yourself in a different light, too. This will illustrate how important your actions are within your world and in turn help you place yourself higher on the scale.

ACTION POINT 3: TRIM AND SWITCH

WHAT YOU NEED TO DO

One of the main barriers to raising yourself up your priority list is often a lack of available time. So, each day, if you find your 'to do' list is longer than five items long, trim it so that you have no more than four tasks outside of work that need to be completed that day. Once you have your four, switch one of them so it is a 'to do' task for you! Build in self-care. Do unto yourself as you would do unto others. Also have a look back at action point 4 in step five. Learning to press the pause button works hand in hand with this action point.

THE LOGIC

Altering your 'to do' list in this way enables you to put into action the thoughts that accompany the notion of prioritizing and valuing yourself. The previous action points may have helped you realize that you are not addressing your own needs. Acknowledging this is the first step, but trimming and switching your daily tasks gives you the opportunity to do something about it and build in some time for you. Make it a habit.

ACTION POINT 4: STICK UP FOR YOURSELF

WHAT YOU NEED TO DO

Learning to stick up for yourself is an important pedestal-climbing skill. Contrary to what many people believe, this doesn't mean you have to become aggressive or confrontational; instead, a good way to start is by expressing yourself constructively. Use 'I' statements instead of focusing on the other person's failings. For example, instead of 'You're so critical', try 'I feel criticized' – you'll make your point without putting the other person on the defensive. If the person still explodes and makes you feel unworthy, avoid caving in and backing down; instead tell them you'll talk when they are ready, then go for a walk, call a friend or pick up a good book. Stand by your feelings, even if it takes some time for them to come round. While talking openly may cost you false relationships it will deepen your genuine ones.

THE LOGIC

If you are low down on your priority list others may start to view you as being less important too. People perceive what you project and will project that back at you – so value yourself, your opinions and your needs and then others will, too.

ACTION POINT 5: LEARN TO SAY NO

WHAT YOU NEED TO DO

It's as simple as it sounds – learn to say no. Practise in front of the mirror; get used to the sound of the word in your mouth. 'No' is a word women don't say often enough – taking on more and more tasks and responsibilities simply because they are asked or expected to. Start by saying no to small things that you don't want to do, or don't realistically have time for, and then build up to more important matters.

THE LOGIC

Ever heard the phrase 'if you want a job done, ask a busy person'? The idea is that the busy person won't turn you down, no matter how many other things they have on their plate. Don't become that busy person that others see as a place to deposit all the stuff they need to get done. Whether it's your boss, your husband, the kids, the in-laws or your mother, learn to say 'no' firmly but nicely and free yourself from chores and commitments that leave you with no space for your own needs and desires.

THE BOTTOM LINE

You don't have to be top of your priority list; it's about balance and developing a symbiotic relationship with yourself, your actions, your family and friends. Once you are standing on your pedestal, you are ready for step seven.

Case study

Making time for yourself is easier said than done. I have found that for many of the highly successful profession-al women and celebrities I see, taking that time out can be just as hard as it is for the rest of us. One particular client, who was on a board of directors, found that the only way she was able to take time out was by booking herself a weekly facial. As luxurious as this sounds, she explained to me that this was the only time when her mobile phone was turned off and she could pay some much-needed time and attention to herself.

Finding and making time for yourself can take many forms. One of my favourite strategies, especially when I am writing my books, is to factor in a duck session! What's a duck session? There's a route near my home that takes me past a duck pond, so as part of my walk I always pack a small bag of stale bread to feed the ducks. I find this simple act very therapeutic and grounding, as it takes me back to the simple pleasures of life. Even if I'm only there for five minutes, I feel so much better. So, whatever does it for you, do try to find that buffer, that small snippet of time when you do something just for you.

STEP SEVEN: FINDING THE ELUSIVE G SPOT

Look along the rows of women's magazines and there will inevitably be numerous articles on sex and at least one that revolves around sexual satisfaction and finding your G spot. Finding your G spot heightens your enjoyment of sex and, naturally, once you enjoy something you start to want more. Finding your G spot is therefore a great motivation for sex.

If you want to drop a size for life you need to find your G spot for weight loss. What is your long-term motivation to keep your weight down? For many, finding their true G spot for weight loss, as in sex, can be difficult. Many of us can fake it and convince ourselves we've found it, giving the equivalent of the Oscar-winning *When Harry met Sally* performance – but we can't keep up the performance forever! Our weight loss G spot can be elusive, but tapping into it is essential if you want to keep that weight off for life.

Weight loss G spots can be big or small. A small G spot may be to lose weight for a summer holiday, a special occasion or maybe your wedding day. Small G spots are short term. If you want to stay at a smaller size for life, you have to find your big G spot.

TYPICAL SMALL G SPOTS

I want to drop a size to …
- wear that string bikini this summer holiday
- look fantastic in a little black dress for the office party
- see my friends again at the school reunion
- lose the 5 pounds I gained over Christmas
- find myself a partner
- look better than the new girlfriend/boyfriend I was dumped for

TYPICAL BIG G SPOTS

I want to drop a size …
- to enjoy better health and energy levels
- to be around to enjoy my children
- for health reasons – one parent died through heart disease/diabetes/stroke, all of which are associated with carrying excess weight
- to increase my chances of avoiding breast cancer, as there is a family history
- to keep fit and well so that I'm able to play with my grandchildren

Don't panic if your G spot starts small, because whatever initially starts you off on your journey to dropping a size for good, is great. However, to keep that momentum throughout your life you will need that big G spot.

Your G spot may, of course, change as you go through your life. When you're younger, getting in shape for a holiday or that date with a special person can be of more significance than your health in later life, as this seems a long way off. So your G spot may be smaller then. However, as you progress through life and your priorities shift, your G spot may naturally get bigger.

Step seven action aims are about finding your true G spot.

ACTION POINT 1: WRITE DOWN YOUR PREVIOUS MOTIVATIONS FOR WANTING TO LOSE WEIGHT

WHAT YOU NEED TO DO

You may have tried every diet in the past – you could wax lyrical about this regime and that regime till the cows come home – but however many you've tried I want you to write down your motivation for each one. Next to this write whether you felt your G spot motivation was a small one or a large one.

THE LOGIC

This enables you to see what motivates you to lose weight and, in the process, it reveals what – and how big – your G spots are. You may find that by adding small G spots together you can create one bigger one.

ACTION POINT 2: IDENTIFY PREVIOUS MOTIVATIONAL MOMENTS

WHAT YOU NEED TO DO

Identify an event or period in the past when have you been really motivated to do something – perhaps it was to get through your professional qualifications, recover from an operation, or plan a surprise party for someone – and you succeeded. Think back to how strongly motivated you were and how you can reach that level of motivation again.

THE LOGIC

If you were strong enough to have the motivation to accomplish those things, then you can equally apply the same level of strength to dropping a size. This action point is about tapping into that motivational strength so that you can use it to help you reach your goal.

ACTION POINT 3: PLAY CUT AND PASTE

WHAT YOU NEED TO DO

This is a simple game that helps you identify how large your G spot is. Make two lists: in the first, make a note of all your bad lifestyle habits; in the second, write down all your good lifestyle habits. (If you have trouble with this you may find it helpful to look at section two, which will give you ideas on how many good and bad habits you have.) Now decide which bad habits you are prepared to cut and which good habits you are prepared to paste over them with. Next, ask yourself how long you are prepared to do this for – is it a day, a week, a fortnight, a month or longer?

THE LOGIC

If you are prepared to cut and paste all of your bad habits for a short period of time this indicates that your motivation is more of a small G spot – you want the gratification, but it looks like it will be short-lived. However, if you find it more comfortable to cut and paste a few of your bad habits with a few good habits and, crucially, keep doing this for a longer period, then you're the lucky owner of a big G spot!

Case study: Kath's Success

Kath was a client who had previously recovered from cancer. Her strength and motivation in aiding her recovery helped her to drop a size and keep it off. Whenever she felt she was heading for an intimate encounter with a gallon of ice cream, she would say to herself 'if I was motivated enough to help myself recover from cancer, I can most definitely be motivated enough not to stuff my face with ice cream'.

Case Study: Ceinwen's Success

'I found university really stressful and ate copious amounts of food as a means of coping. Over 3½ years I put on 30kg. No matter how hard I tried to motivate myself, the stress of studying won. Then I saw a TV documentary about a woman who lost the same amount of weight in 40 weeks as part of a bet she made with a public betting agency. I decided to make the same bet myself – to lose 30kg and keep it off for 12 months. This gave me the motivation I needed and I followed the carb curfew eating plan, incorporating tips from slimming magazines, books and clubs. I now weigh 73kg and will lose another 5kg over the next few months while I finish my degree.'

THE BOTTOM LINE

Our motivation for doing something can change throughout life – the important thing is to know what your motivation is and for your reasons to be as compelling as possible. The bigger your weight loss G spot, the more ways you are likely to be able to stimulate it.

By now you should be the right space to drop a size – so let's move on to the really practical stuff.

DROPPING
THAT SIZE

INTRODUCTION

To drop a size you have to have willpower, but to stay at that size you need to learn how to steer your new relationship between your body and brain through a series of challenges. If you want to drop a size and stay at your new size for life you will need to learn how to navigate your day, your week, your month, and your year − in all its seasonal guises. To enable you to do just that this section features a variety of eating and exercise plans for you to choose from. These work hand in hand with the 10 foolproof principles − I call them fundamentals − that underpin the Drop a Size for Life plan. In this section, you'll also find a list of foods and recipe ideas that will keep you in top health, whether you're losing weight or maintaining your weight loss.

Case Study: Jonathan's Success

'It's the only plan I have ever done (and I have done lots!) where after one year I weigh less than I did at the end of the course − it's a very simple plan that is easy to maintain and causes little disruption.' Jonathan lost 13kg/28½lb and dropped three sizes.

The truth is that although many of us think we know what a healthy diet entails, we are often wide of the mark, or not as up-to-date as we might think. For example, the classic food pyramid, with starchy carbohydrates forming the base, is now being widely criticized by physicians, researchers and dieters, because it doesn't distinguish between highly refined carbohydrates, such as white flour and rice, and healthier wholegrains like brown rice or wholemeal pasta and bread. The first step in this section is therefore to get your head around the 10 fundamentals – these combine the basics of a healthy diet with my strategies for losing weight and keeping it off.

Case Study: Emma's Success

'Due to the nature of my business I wasn't able to take the time to make up all the recipes, so I had to be flexible. I was never hungry but felt very nourished. My advice would be not to lose heart if you can't follow all the recipes. Just follow the fundamentals and you will succeed. It worked for me and I was thrilled at the change in body shape above all. This is the only diet that has ever worked for me.' Emma lost 2.7kg/6lb and dropped a size.

THE 10 FUNDAMENTALS

FOLLOW THE CARB CURFEW

My Carb Curfew means, quite simply, cutting out the starchy carbs after 5 p.m. It is the single most important factor in my clients' weight management success – in their own words.

Case Study: Jane's Success

'If you only do one thing, give up the carbs after 5 p.m. While I initially only experienced a small weight reduction, the effect became apparent after a year, due almost entirely to Joanna's no starchy carbs after 5 p.m. rule.' Jane lost 5kg/11lb and dropped a size.

The simple act of saying no to starchy carbohydrates like potatoes, rice, pasta, bread and cereals after 5 p.m. has three main benefits:

1. **It cuts down calories without the need for calorie counting**

   By cutting out starchy carbohydrates after 5 p.m. you will naturally be cutting your calorie intake. However, since you'll be filling up on more fruit and vegetables, lean meat, fish and energy-providing pulses, you won't feel hungry.

2. **It boosts your energy**

   Excess starch stimulates the production of serotonin in the brain, which can make us feel more sluggish. Eating a lighter meal based on protein, vegetables and fruit will provide more energy and keep your energy levels steady. As an added bonus, eating more fruit and vegetables will boost your intake of essential vitamins and minerals.

3. **It reduces bloating**

   Excess starch intake can leave you feeling heavy and bloated. That's because for every unit of glycogen (the storage form that carbohydrate takes in the body), you need three units of water with which to store it. Think of it this way: if you eat a cereal bowl-sized portion of pasta your body has to hold onto three bowls of water to be able to convert the starch to glycogen to be stored. That's not to say we don't need glycogen – it is an essential fuel – but we can only store a limited amount and if we do not burn it through regular exercise, it will be converted and stored as fat.

Having dispensed with the starchy carbohydrates, your evening meal should now be based around vegetables; protein-providing lean meats, pulses and fish; some essential fats and fruit. You can have some dairy products, too. It may take you a little time to get used to this way of eating but once you have you'll be amazed by the results and how simple it is to apply. You'll find lots of ideas for Carb Curfew recipes on pages 196–237.

WHY DO WE NEED CARBOHYDRATES?

Carbohydrates provide the energy, in the form of glucose, needed for all the cellular processes that take place in the body. The right carbs also prevent the all too common 'brain freeze' that can occur when our blood sugar gets too low and we get fuzzy-headed. Although the body can break down fat and protein for energy, this takes time so a steady stream of glucose from the right carbs is your brain's preferred fuel. Carbs also provide essential vitamins and minerals, which, together with healthy plant phytochemicals found in tomatoes, dark green vegetables and orange and yellow fruit and veg, work together to fight cancer, heart disease and Alzheimer's disease.

However, not all carbohydrates work in the same way, especially in terms of the way they affect blood glucose levels. This has an important bearing on your efforts to drop a size, as learning how to control your blood glucose levels is crucial to feeling energized, and helping prevent cravings and overeating.

THE DIFFERENT CARBOHYDRATES

I've talked a lot about carbohydrates, but what exactly is a carbohydrate? Well the scientific answer is it's an organic compound containing carbon, hydrogen and oxygen – but that's of little practical use to us. Of more interest is the fact that carbs are generally classified as simple or complex. Simple carbohydrates provide instant but not long-lasting energy. Examples of simple carbs include sugars and starches found in sweets, cakes, biscuits and some fruits. Simple carbs cause a surge of insulin, which ultimately causes blood sugar levels to drop. This drop alerts the brain to issue hunger signals in an attempt to get some glucose to fuel it. These hunger signals often result in overeating or eating additional calories that your body, from an energy balance perspective, doesn't actually need.

In contrast, complex carbohydrates are released into the bloodstream more slowly and therefore take longer to digest. Examples include most fruits, vegetables and high-fibre, wholemeal breads. In general, complex carbohydrates have less impact on blood glucose and insulin levels and are less likely to be stored as fat.

The answer then is to eat more fruit and vegetables and fewer simple carbohydrates. Unfortunately, many of us eat far too many carbohydrates, especially the simple ones. Therefore, as well as operating the Carb Curfew as a simple means of eating less carbs, we also need to remember to eat the right type of carbs! If you eat too many refined carbs, such as bread, pittas and refined rice and pasta, you will raise your blood sugar sky high and this drastic rise in glucose will create a larger production of insulin. And when you combine excess carb calories with insulin your body becomes more receptive to storing these as fat.

In addition, decades of research confirms that eating a diet high in fruit, vegetables and wholegrains lowers your risk of cancer, prevents disease and promotes longevity – so any diet that restricts these food groups too stringently should be suspect.

WHY CERTAIN CARBS ARE BAD FOR YOUR HEALTH

Eating a diet high in refined carbohydrates may put women at risk of two kinds of cancer. Looking at data from the 18-year Nurses' Health Study, National Cancer Institute researchers found that sedentary, overweight women who ate diets high in added sugar and white flour had a 53 per cent increased risk of pancreatic cancer, which has a five year survival rate of only four per cent. Another study looked at the diets of more than 2,500 Italian women with breast cancer and an equal number who were cancer-free and found that the women with breast cancer ate more foods high in refined carbs. Foods such as white bread and cookies boost blood sugar and insulin levels, while triggering a rise in the insulin-like growth hormones that are linked to breast cancer risk.

In both studies, researchers discovered that the women's diets included a significant number of foods with a high Glycaemic index (GI) and Glycaemic load (GL).

MAKING CARBS WORK FOR YOU

The GI concept has been around for quite some time. It is a measurement of how fast and how high blood sugar and insulin rise after a form of carbohydrate is eaten. It sounds simple enough but it can be misleading. For example, both white bread and carrots have high GI numbers of 70 and 71 respectively, suggesting that they both send blood sugar soaring. However, that's true only if you eat more than 625g of carrots, compared with just four slices of white bread! Now that is a lot of carrots.

The Glycaemic load, in comparison, is much more practical and user-friendly, as it measures the effect on blood sugar of a normal serving of food. Using this method, the GL for two slices of white bread turns out to be more than five times higher than the GL for ½ cup of carrots.

By accounting for serving size, the new GL method helps in choosing foods to control blood glucose and consequently insulin levels. You'll find the GL concept, used in conjunction with the Carb Curfew, is not only beneficial in helping control your size – it could also help prevent cancer and control diabetes.

To keep blood glucose from peaking, minimize your intake of foods with a high GL, such as white flour and sugar. To keep blood glucose moderate, maximize foods with a low GL, such as fruits, veg and grains. And operating my carb curfew is one of the simplest ways to do this.

A comparison of GI and GL for some common foods appears below. Although there is no consensus yet on what is a high, medium or low GL, the spread of numbers across the spectrum of foodstuffs suggests that above 20 is high, between 10 and 20 is medium and below 10 is low.

Food	Glycaemic Index (GI)	Glycaemic Load (GL)
Instant rice	91	24.8
Baked potato	85	20.3
Cornflakes	84	21
Carrots	71	3.8
White bread	70	21
Rye bread	65	19.5
Muesli	56	16.8
Banana	53	13.3
Spaghetti	41	16.4
Apple	36	8.1
Lentils	29	5.7
Milk	27	3.2
Peanuts	27	0.7

Note: Most non-starchy vegetables have values too low to measure and are therefore classed as low GL foods.

When eating a meal made up of a combination of different food groups, bear in mind that the rate of glucose released into the bloodstream will be affected by all the foods eaten. For example, protein and fibre – and acid-based dressings such as vinegar – all slow the rate of blood glucose release.

SOME COMMON QUESTIONS

Should I cut out all carbs?

The simple answer is NO! As we have seen, carbohydrates are present in fruits, vegetables and wholegrains, as well as in processed foods such as sweets, cakes and biscuits. If you were to cut all carbs from your diet you would be depriving your body of the essential minerals and vitamins provided by fruit and vegetables, as well as essential dietary fibre from wholegrains. The quantity of carbs we eat does need to be cut down, but cutting out all carbs forces the body into a condition known as ketosis, where an abnormal build up of substances called ketones creates a situation of false starvation in the body. When the body does not have enough glucose (from carbohydrate) for fuel it relies on an imperfect back-up system that utilizes protein and fat for energy. Ketosis causes the body to kick into starvation mode, even to the point of leaching the calcium from your bones.

Help! How can I follow the Carb Curfew when I eat at restaurants virtually all the time?

Putting the Carb Curfew into practice really is a breeze when it comes to eating out at restaurants. Even good ol' spaghetti-loving Italian restaurants will always offer at least one meat- or fish-orientated dish without pasta. And if your meal does arrive with pasta or rice you can leave it to one side. My clients tell me that knowing in advance that they're going to order a starch-free meal from the menu really helps their diet choice. They're confident that they're making the best choice for their health and size, without having to puzzle over the prospective fat grams or calories. In addition, if you feel more comfortable not telling people you are following a healthy diet plan, no one need know because your meal selection will appear perfectly normal. Cutting the carbs is a simple and enjoyable way of eating and one that puts the pleasure back into eating out.

How do I cope with going to a friend's house for dinner?

If you're not sure whether or not you'll be able to avoid the carbs, don't panic! I find the best way to deal with this is to switch your Carb Curfew meal time to your lunch or breakfast – making these what I call carb-free zones. That way you will have freed up your carb option, so if a plate of pasta is served you can enjoy it without feeling you have blown the Carb Curfew. Making your breakfast or lunch a carb-free zone gives you flexibility when you need it – however, I would still encourage you to operate the Carb Curfew rule after 5 p.m. whenever possible. This has the greatest success with my clients, partly because it helps them control their calorie intake without much thought, and at a time of day when our willpower is naturally low. In addition, going to bed and waking up not feeling bloated is a huge catalyst to help you feel better in your self – not to mention the fact that it makes you feel as if you've already dropped a size!

How can I follow the Carb Curfew when I work night shifts?

Working shifts can have a huge impact on your meals, meal times and energy levels. Many nurses and long-haul air stewards have found the following advice a great help.

Before you go to work (probably late afternoon or early evening) have a light meal containing some carbohydrate, protein and fat. Selecting low to moderate GL carbohydrates, such as pulses, fruit and vegetables, together with some protein, will give you a slow release of energy through the first part of your evening shift. I have found with my clients that it helps to think of this meal as your 'breakfast' so have a look at the breakfast suggestions on pages 190–192 for ideas.

In the middle of your shift (generally around midnight to 1 a.m.) have your Carb Curfew meal of protein, vegetables, fruit and essential fats. The protein will stimulate the production of the brain transmitter dopamine, which will boost your feelings of alertness at a time when you may be feeling a little jaded. Do avoid too large a meal at this time, as eating a meal containing more than 1000 calories in one go has been shown to bring on feelings of sleepiness and lethargy. Have a snack around 4 or 5 a.m., such as a glass of semi or skimmed milk and a small cube of dark chocolate (yes you can eat chocolate on my diet plan!). This may feel like a real reward, but the health-giving phenols found in dark chocolate can actually improve your cholesterol levels (if eaten in small amounts) and improve the elasticity of your blood vessels. The sweetness of the chocolate will also give you a bit of a buzz, while the milk is a great source of calcium and protein and will hydrate you and stretch your stomach lining, helping you to feel full. (You'll find more snack ideas on page 194.) When you get home, and before you go to bed, you may want to have a light meal containing a little starch, protein and fat. A poached egg on a slice of wholemeal toast plus a couple of grilled tomatoes, or a bowl of wholegrain cereal are good options. They're easy to digest, not too calorific and will give you a feeling of satisfaction before you go to sleep.

THE BOTTOM LINE – WHAT YOU NEED TO DO

- Operate my Carb Curfew.
- Select carbs with a low to moderate GL at breakfast and lunch.
- Use carb-free zones when you are unsure what will be available for your evening meal.

EAT MORE FIBRE

We simply do not get enough fibre in our diets and, with the current popularity of high protein diets, our intake of dietary fibre is believed to be falling further. More and more people are cutting out wholegrains from their diet, leaving a big fibre deficit and depriving themselves of this essential dietary component. A high-fibre diet is the right choice for many reasons: it can give your energy levels a boost and it helps lower the risk of diabetes, heart disease and bowel cancer – and, of course, it aids regular bowel movements.

If your diet is 'average', you are probably eating around 13g or less of fibre a day. In the UK, the relevant authorities suggest that adults should aim for an average of 18g a day for protective health benefits. However, the US Food and Nutrition Board recently set the first recommended daily intakes and these are much higher: they suggest that men up to age 50 require 38g of fibre daily, while women need 25g; men and women over 50 should get 30g and 21g respectively.

In order to achieve the US recommended daily intake, you would need to eat a minimum of six servings of fruit and veg and three servings of wholegrains daily. It might sound a lot, but since fibre slows digestion and makes you feel full, it may aid your weight loss efforts, as well as improving your general health. A word of warning: it will probably take your system a number of days to adjust to a higher fibre level, but do stay with it. You may experience some stomach discomfort and bloating at first, but during the second week you should feel an improvement. It will stave off hunger and your health will definitely benefit.

Fibre comes in two forms, soluble and insoluble. Soluble fibre dissolves in water and forms a gel – it is found in fruits, vegetables, legumes (pulses such as beans) and oat bran, and can help reduce cholesterol when eaten as part of a diet low in saturated fat. Soluble fat can also help control blood sugar. Insoluble fibre cannot dissolve in water, but instead absorbs water as it passes through the body. Found in fruits, vegetables, whole grains and wheat bran, it adds faecal bulk and helps speed up the rate at which food passes through the digestive system.

HOW TO INCREASE YOUR FIBRE INTAKE

A single bowl of high-fibre cereal is a great way to get more fibre and, if you're a cereal eater, you can do some simple swaps to boost your fibre intake. See the chart on pages 96–97 for some ideas.

Does this tickle your G spot?

People who eat a high-fibre breakfast cereal tend to feel more energetic than those who eat low-fibre cereals. They also report feeling better and even thinking more clearly. It's thought that this is in part explained by the fact that eating high-fibre cereals alleviates that little problem that no one really likes to talk about – constipation, and hence leaves people feeling lighter and more comfortable. Fatigue is extremely prevalent in our society so if increasing your fibre intake boosts your energy, it's a great incentive to eat more of it.

'I personally favour a high-fibre supplement as I find this the easiest way to get fibre into my diet. It means I don't have to rummage around in the supermarket trying to find not only the sandwich filling I like, but also the right type of bread. I grind flax seeds or buy Fibroflax, a combination of flaxseed, psyllium husk and anti-ageing vitamin E-rich wheatgerm. I add it to my cereal, smoothies, yoghurt, fruit, soups – in fact just about anything that I can sprinkle it on.'

Joanna

SIMPLE BREAKFAST FIBRE MAKEOVERS

Your current breakfast	Total Fibre	Total Calories
50g Cheerios with 125ml skimmed milk and 1 glass orange juice	3.25g	326
50g Special K with 125ml skimmed milk and 1 piece white toasted bread with jam	1.7g	334
50g Cornflakes with 125ml skimmed milk and a small banana	2g	297
50g Crunchy Nut Cornflakes with 125ml skimmed milk and 125g strawberries	3.5g	257

How to increase your fibre intake	Total Fibre	Total Calories
Replace the orange juice with prune juice and you'll increase your fibre intake by 2g; replace the Cheerios with Shreddies and you increase it by a further 2g	7.25g	371
Replace Special K with Bran Flakes with Fruits and you'll increase your fibre intake by 4.5g. Replacing white bread with wholemeal will add another 1g of fibre and having peanut butter instead of jam will add another 2g	9.2g	375
Have only 25g of Cornflakes and replace the other 25g with 25g of All Bran – this will increase your fibre intake by 7.2g	9.2g	262
Replace the Crunchy Nut Cornflakes with Crunchy Oat Bran with Fruits to add another 4g of fibre. Sprinkle 15g pumpkin seeds on the strawberries to add a further 2.1g of fibre	9.6g	298

Looks can be deceiving

Which do you think has the most fibre – a stick of celery or half an avocado? Believe it or not, the avocado has the most. Looks and tastes can be deceiving, so use this list of high-fibre foods (defined as those containing at least 5g of fibre per serving) as a guide.

- Apples, plums, pears
- Beans (dried and fresh), peas and other legumes, including chickpeas and lentils
- Blackberries, blueberries and raspberries
- Broccoli
- Cherries
- Corn
- Dried fruits, particularly apricots, dates and figs
- Greens, including kale, spinach and Swiss chard
- Nuts, especially almonds, Brazil nuts and walnuts
- Wholegrains, such as whole-wheat pasta, bulgur wheat and bran cereals

THE BOTTOM LINE – WHAT YOU NEED TO DO

- Introduce a combination of soluble and insoluble fibre into your daily diet.
- Get off to a good start and fibre-fortify your breakfast either with a suitable cereal or supplement.
- Gently and gradually introduce more fibre into your diet so it is not a sudden shock to your system!

CUT YOUR SODIUM INTAKE

Salt is the name we give to the mineral sodium chloride. It looks harmless enough and it adds taste without calories – but it may just be sabotaging your weight loss efforts. I will admit there is scant scientific evidence to support the role of sodium in weight loss, however, I have observed time and time again that simply getting clients to switch from a high-salt diet to a low-salt diet brings significant weight loss results. Admittedly, they are consuming fewer calories, but the amount of weight loss and inch loss is far greater than could be attributed to calorie reduction alone. More research is required here, but it appears that some people are more sodium sensitive than others – which means their bodies hold onto more water and as a result they feel puffy and bloated. I have seen this specifically in overweight clients, where puffiness and swelling directly affects their quality and freedom of movement.

Does this tickle your G spot?

If you like a drink or two as well as your salt, then this could affect your sodium sensitivity. Research conducted at the School of Medicine, University of Buffalo, suggests that chronic heavy alcohol intake increases sodium sensitivity. So think twice before you order your third pint and packet of salted peanuts! You can find out more about alcohol and weight loss on pages 171–174.

While we know that sodium may not contribute to the size of your fat cells, it can affect your dress size by causing fluid retention. This not only has a bearing on how you feel physically in your body, but it can also make you feel uncomfortable and push you further away from being in the right space to drop a size.

If you don't routinely sprinkle salt on your food, you may think this isn't an issue for you – however, we're not just talking about the salt shaker here. Sodium finds its way into our diet from numerous processed foods. A pre-prepared carton of beef stew, for example, can contain up to 6g of salt, while canned soup may have up to 3g of salt per can. A slice of bread gives us 0.4g of salt per slice and 25g of Cheddar cheese a further 0.4g. In fact, the amount of salt is so high in many of the processed and packaged foods we buy – including not just the obvious things such as crisps and nuts, but also biscuits, breakfast cereals and canned vegetables – that the Food Standards Agency is lobbying the food industry to reduce added salt.

We do need a certain amount of sodium for our bodies to function – to keep nerve pathways working, to regulate fluid balance and to maintain our muscles – but too much salt has been clearly linked with hypertension (it raises blood pressure), which in turn increases the risk of heart disease or stroke, two of Britain's biggest killers. Government guidelines recommend consuming no more than 4g of salt a day (4g of salt contains 1600mg of sodium) – that's the equivalent of a level teaspoon. Research suggests we are potentially shaking on 9g a day – so we would do well to look for alternative ways of flavouring our food. Try seasoning the foods you cook with spices, herbs, lemon and salt-free seasoning blends and, as the stuff we shake over our food contributes just 20 per cent of the sodium in the typical British diet, avoid processed foods that are high in salt.

You might also like to try reduced-sodium salt (such as Lo-Salt); this contains potassium chloride in place of some of the sodium and only has a third of the sodium content of standard table salt. Natural sea salt by comparison is also healthier, since it contains many minerals, including magnesium and calcium.

Case Study: Chris's Success

When Chris first came to me on ITV's *This Morning* he was unable to sleep at night without the aid of a special tube to keep his throat open. He found walking quite painful and he looked very puffy and way older than his 42 years. Chris told me he had tried many diets in the past but had never been able to stick to them or found they just didn't work. Instead of asking Chris to cut his calories, I asked him to do just three things:

- Switch from a high-salt diet to a low-salt diet.
- Operate the Carb Curfew.
- Eat more potassium-rich vegetables to help stabilize his high salt intake.

'Switching my diet from a high salt one to a low salt one seemed so much easier and appealing than cutting calories and not eating some of my favourite foods. All I had to do was make a few switches between what I normally picked when I was on the road driving my truck. At the end of just one week I had lost 11 pounds – I was amazed! The biggest difference was how I was able to move my body – I had so much more movement in all my joints that I wanted to get out and walk, whereas before walking had always caused my joints to hurt. After two weeks I had dropped a stone. How simple was that! Joanna explained to me that my loss was not all body fat and most of it was fluid, but it gave me the impetus to keep going. My body felt so much better, I was sleeping better and I stopped needing the tube at night to keep my throat open.' So Chris was a real success, he lost 11kg/24lb. He knows he still has some way to go, but making that simple change to his diet has allowed him to be so much more physically active.

As I stated earlier, I'm not trying to claim reducing sodium is the latest weight loss tool — it isn't. But, without doubt, some people are more sodium sensitive than others and fluid retention can account for some of their extra inches. This can make people feel even more uncomfortable about their weight and push them further away from being in the right space to drop a size. So see sodium reduction as a path to better health and a way of feeling more comfortable in and with your body.

Does this tickle your G spot?

Halving salt intake in the UK could save 34,000 lives a year, according to one recent report. It would also be sufficient to significantly reduce blood pressure in those suffering from hypertension. Eating too much salt has also been linked to osteoporosis and stomach cancer.

Who gains the most from cutting their salt?

I have found that clients who are over 40, lead a sedentary lifestyle and have a cluster of conditions, such as high blood pressure, insulin resistance and a family history of diabetes, stand to gain the most from decreasing their sodium intake. This clustering of conditions is known as Metabolic Syndrome X or Insulin Resistance Syndrome. You can read more about this on page 338.

Certain groups of people – namely the elderly, African-Americans and those with a family history of high blood pressure – are also more likely to have blood pressure that's particularly salt (or sodium) sensitive.

HIDDEN SALT

You may not use a salt shaker but hidden sodium can lurk in many everyday foods. We only need 4g a day – remember that's the equivalent of a level teaspoon. The fact is that there's so much salt in normal foodstuffs that it is easy to eat double that amount without knowing it. Sprinkling salt on your food or using salt when cooking vegetables can easily add another 2g to your daily total. The typical daily diets listed opposite show how easy it is to overload on salt (the salt counts are for the content of the meals *before* any extra seasoning is added):

Breakfast: Cornflakes (50g, 1.4g salt) and milk, 2 slices of toast with salted butter (1.2g) and marmalade
Lunch: BLT sandwich (2 slices bread, 2.5g), orange drink, packet of crisps (0.5g), apple
Dinner: Chicken and vegetable stir-fry (with 115g chicken, 180g mixed veg and 1 tbsp soy sauce, 3.2g salt), yoghurt, cheese (55g Cheddar, 1g salt) and biscuits (4 salted cracker-type biscuits, 1.2g)
TOTAL: 11g salt = 2.2 teaspoons

Breakfast: Porridge (0.25g per bowl), 2 slices of toast with salted butter (1.2g) and Marmite
Lunch: Big Mac and large fries (3.5g salt)
Dinner: Ready-made supermarket lasagne (up to 4.5g salt), spinach salad
TOTAL: 9.4g salt = 1.9 teaspoons

Breakfast: Bagel (0.5g) with 2oz salmon (1.7g) and cream cheese (0.1g)
Lunch: Noodle snack (100g, about 4.5g)
Dinner: Ready-made soup (3g), 85g wholemeal bread (1.26g), bread-crumbed fish steak (1g), potatoes, broccoli
TOTAL: 12.1g salt = 2.4 teaspoons

Breakfast: Bacon (2 rashers, 1.8g salt), eggs, sausage (two, 1.8g), baked beans (1.25g per serving), 1 slice of toast with salted butter (0.6g)

Pub lunch: peanuts (small packet, 0.6g), ploughman's with 100g Stilton (2g salt), 1 tbsp pickle (0.5g) and salad
Dinner: Home-cooked paella containing chorizo sausage, prawns (2.7g), green salad, poached pears in red wine, with cream (0.25g)
TOTAL: 11.5g salt = 2.3 teaspoons

HOW TO MEASURE HOW MUCH SALT YOU ARE EATING

Some food companies list the amount of sodium in their food products – well done! However, the amount of sodium is not the same as the amount of salt. To work out how much salt the sodium quantity equates to, simply multiply the amount of sodium by 2.5.

Here's an example of a food label:

Typical Values per pack
Energy Kcal: 230
Sodium g: 0.92

The equivalent amount of salt will therefore be 2.3g ($0.92 \times 2.5 = 2.3$g)

The recommendation is that we eat *no more* than 5g daily, therefore this one food item would provide nearly half of that daily limit. Interestingly, this food label is not from a packet of smoked bacon or bag of ready salted crisps but it is from a pre-packed three bean salad – which you wouldn't generally consider as a salty food. So it pays to read your labels and get sodium savvy!

HOW TO CUT BACK ON SODIUM WITHOUT TRYING

1. Eat more foods that contain potassium – fruits, vegetables, lentils, pulses, fresh meat and fish, eggs, unsalted nuts, potatoes, pasta and rice. Potassium balances the effect of salt on the body.
2. Try to avoid processed, cured or pickled foods such as bacon, gammon, sausages, canned meat, packet soups, soy sauce, ketchup or chutneys, crisps, salted or roasted nuts and cheese biscuits. Also avoid fast food, such as hamburgers and chips, which may be very salty. You do need to live your life, so obviously it will be impossible to leave these out of your diet completely, but choose them less often.
3. Don't add table salt to food once it is served.
4. Choose items with reduced sodium content.
5. Monitor the salt content of processed food.
6. Avoid all foods that have more than 0.2g of sodium per 100g. Generally, all packaged foods have added salt but if the sodium content per 100g is greater than 0.2g, the food is high in salt.
7. Instead of salt, use spices and flavourings that are low in salt.
8. In restaurants, choose low-sodium menu items and ask that they prepare your meal without salt or MSG (monosodium glutamate) which, like salt, can raise blood pressure.

THE BOTTOM LINE – WHAT YOU NEED TO DO

- Get sodium savvy and learn the sodium and salt content of the foods you eat most often.
- Eat plenty of vegetables to provide potassium, which helps counteract excess sodium.
- Switch to 'low' salt or sea salt to optimize the minerals your body can use.

FIT IN SOME EXERCISE – WITH AND WITHOUT YOUR TRAINERS

Exercise seems to be the weight-loss fundamental that most people are adverse to. Yet, with just a little effort, it can actually be one of the easiest to fulfil. Admittedly, when it comes to short-term weight loss, what you put in your mouth has a greater impact than exercise – but, in the long term, if you want to keep your weight down, there's no getting away from the fact that physical activity and exercise have to play a regular part in your life.

The number one reason many people cite for not taking regular exercise is lack of time. Step six in section one stressed the importance of taking time to do things for you, but fitting in exercise and physical activity can be a challenge. For this reason, I've provided ways for you to burn energy without having to put your trainers on, as well as structured exercise sessions that you can fit into your day. I call these workout wedges. Finding a workout wedge that's suitable for you and learning how to be more physically active throughout your day is invaluable in helping you drop a size for life.

Does this tickle your G spot?

A recent study, which looked into energy expenditure among women who had lost weight in the previous year, found that the single distinguishing feature between women who had successfully kept their weight off and those who had regained the pounds was physical activity. The energy expenditure among the maintainers was a staggering 44 per cent higher than the women who had gained weight. But don't panic – the maintainers didn't spend half their lives in the gym – some of the activities they did included walking, gardening and stair climbing. That's where physical activity differs from structured exercise – it simply means injecting more energy-burning activity into your day, in any way you can.

Many people are terrified at the prospect of having to join a gym. Gyms are fantastic, but they're not for everyone. You may feel intimidated, you may find they're too expensive, you don't like the classes or the environment, or there isn't one near you … Well you'll be glad to hear it doesn't matter! I have found time and time again with my clients that when life gets busy, the first thing that gets dropped is the regular gym session. So relying too heavily on the gym as your mode of burning calories can actually lull you into a false sense of security. The good news is that you can burn off the same number of calories (or more) as you would in a one-hour aerobics class without ever setting foot in a gym or slipping on your Lycra. How? Well it's something you've probably done at one time or another, but the problem is it never became a long-term habit.

Do you remember a time when you always got up to change the TV channel, you walked to the shops, mowed the lawn – and these sorts of physical activities were all part of your daily life? These are just a few tasks that are becoming obsolete and as a result we are being deprived of everyday physical activity. If you add up all the calories you could burn from just doing a few things that involve actually moving your body, experts have proposed that you could lose up to 38 pounds in one year! It sounds too good to be true, but if you really put your mind to it, you can achieve significant weight loss by just moving more and being creative with how you live your life.

One of the major reasons people are getting heavier is the daily decrease in the amount of physical activity we are doing. The Cooper Institute in America estimates that the average adult expends about 300–700 calories less each day than their parents' generation did. Let's put this into perspective: if you put your body in a 700-calorie gaining situation for five consecutive days, then theoretically, you could gain a pound in weight. This figure is alarming. However, adding activity back into your daily life is an easy and effective way to shape up and slim down.

Relying solely on the gym as your source of exercise is not a successful long-term option. One study compared daily energy expenditure between gym-goers and those who were simply active on a daily basis (walking and cycling, for example) and found that the latter burned more energy and achieved greater health benefits. Gym-goers, it seemed, were more likely to mentally 'tick off' exercise, once they'd done it, and be even more sedentary during the rest of their waking hours. So it pays to navigate your way through your day, building in as much physical activity as you can.

NAVIGATING THE 24

If you have read any of my books before, you'll know I am a firm believer in navigating your 24 hours imaginatively. Think about it: there are 24 hours in the day, approximately nine of which will be used for sleeping – that leaves 15 hours when we can be physically moving our bodies and expending energy. However, 10 of those hours may be used up at work, or with the family, when we may be exhausted by mental strain but not usually by physical activity. For example, we may be sitting in an office dealing with problems that require a lot of mental energy, or we may be dashing around doing school runs, the supermarket food shop and various other errands in the car. The remaining five hours may be used up social-izing, meeting friends and catching up with everyday household chores. Our lives may be very full, but if only 30 minutes of our weekly schedule involves physical exer-tion then dieting alone won't make much difference. Without accumulating our physical activity, when we come to do our structured exercise session not only do we need to burn enough calories in that session to cancel out any excess calories we've eaten, but we also need to make up for the calories we have not been able to burn through-out the day. This means that we are expecting a lot from our one structured exercise session.

So accumulating physical activity during the day is a vital strategy, not only for long-term successful weight and body fat management but also for overall good health. Studies have shown conclusively, for example, that brisk walking at intermittent times during the day has a protec-tive effect against heart disease, diabetes and high blood cholesterol levels. So go on … be active!

Modern society offers so many labour-saving devices that it's very easy for us to become lazy. If we were using all this extra time we're saving ourselves to do something physical, like taking long walks or riding a bike, then that would be great – but in reality that is just not happening. Instead, the vast majority of us – around 54 per cent – don't exercise, and, even if we do, few of us do it regular-ly enough to reap the benefits.

The harsh reality is that many people do not realize how inactive they are. We tell ourselves that because we are busy, we work, we have homes, friends, deadlines, busy social lives, and family to look after that we're pretty active. Yet few of these things involve exerting ourselves physically.

Because time is so precious, it's vital to find an exercise that's easy to fit into your day – and one of the easiest is walking. In fact, navigating your 24 hours so that it includes more walking is fundamental for dropping a size for life.

WALKING

Not only is walking convenient and inexpensive – all you need is a good pair of shoes – but almost anybody can do it and at just about any stage in life. This makes walking the perfect life-long exercise partner. It also has the lowest drop-out rate of any form of exercise.

Studies have shown that walking for just 30 minutes a day can reduce your risk of dying prematurely and of developing numerous chronic diseases. In addition, it will control your weight, build and maintain healthy muscle tissue, bones and joints, and boost your mood. Many people approach exercise with an 'all or nothing' attitude, which means they either go all out at the gym or are a complete couch potato. However, we can start to challenge this approach to exercise by making walking the backbone of our drop a size for life strategy. Walking with a little thought can become such an integral part of our life again that we can make all our activities aerobic, calorie-burning opportunities without even realizing – even shopping can become aerobic!

Vote with your feet

If there's one sound investment the government could make for the nation's health it would be to give every single adult a pedometer. These easy to use, inexpensive devices measure the number of steps you take each day and I've no doubt they would convince many people of their inactivity and jolt them into action! Studies have shown you need to take a minimum of 4000 steps a day to impact on your health and 10,000 a day for weight management. More recent studies conducted in the US have shown individuals lost weight when they walked 17,500 steps a day, despite making no changes to their diet. Considering that a recent report estimated obesity costs the NHS £2.8 billion each year, I think a pedometer per adult would be sound economic management.

EIGHT SIMPLE WAYS TO NAVIGATE YOUR 24

1. Take your foot off cruise control

   Increase the intensity of your everyday activities, whether you're vacuuming or walking the dog. Turn on some music with an energizing beat to help keep the tempo up, or

invest in a music-playing pedometer, which plays a tune as
you walk and speeds up the tune the faster you walk.

2. Step up and down

Stairs are great leg strengtheners. Lifting you body against
gravity is one of the best ways to burn calories, while the
impact of stepping downstairs can protect against a loss
of bone density. So try to take the stairs at every
opportunity – even on moving escalators always resolve
to walk up them. While standing at the bus stop, why not
step up and down off the kerb?

3. Burn calories as you stand

Poor posture means you are burning fewer calories – so
by standing tall you not only look thinner, but you're also
burning more calories. To help you with your posture,
imagine you have to hold a pencil between your shoulder
blades and, at the same time, be able to slip your fingertips
inside your waistband and carry a book on your head.
Visualizing these three simple things will automatically
improve your posture.

4. Make your bags your dumbbells

Every time you let someone else pack your shopping,
carry your bags, or load your car, you're depriving your
body of the opportunity to enhance your muscle mass
and burn vital calories. You don't have to be a martyr and
carrying too heavy a load can be detrimental to you, but if
you're capable of doing it then do it. Try to evenly load
bags so you can carry a bag of equal weight in each hand
and, when travelling, pack two small suitcases or holdalls –

one big suitcase is hard to carry and you'll need to twist
your spine to lift it effectively.

5. Park your bum on a ball

   Replace your office chair with a Swiss ball. These large
   inflated balls are not only comfortable but are a great way
   to challenge your core abdominal muscles as you sit.
   Sitting in a normal chair can make these muscles become
   lazy as they stop doing the important job of supporting
   the spine. When muscles stop contracting they burn
   fewer calories – admittedly the number of extra calories
   burnt will not be great, but done day in day out they
   all add up.

6. Go the distance

   Make a short list of a few things you do each day that you
   can work a bit of exercise into. For example, if you work
   in an office, one of the simplest things you can do is start
   using the loo on the floor above – taking the stairs of
   course. Park your car at the far end of the supermarket
   car park and not as close as you can get it. These may
   seem like small things but done regularly you will be surprised how they impact on your weight loss and fitness.
   Finding the longest route can be a great habit to get into
   – and no one will know what you're doing.

7. Do chair-robics

   Set your timer to go off every hour and get up off your
   chair and do four squats. It's a great way to boost
   circulation, thus aiding cellulite reduction and boosting
   oxygen to your skin, which helps you to look younger and

fresher. It will also give you a gentle stretch. Four squats
every hour – that's all I'm asking for!

8. Mind the gap

   Don't just sit there while you're waiting for the kettle to
   boil or your email to download, get up, stretch, walk
   around, complete another task. Perform a few buttock
   squeezes. All these small things do make a difference. You'll
   find other helpful ideas for filling those gap moments in
   the section below.

HOW ABOUT A WORKOUT WEDGE?

What's a workout wedge? A workout wedge is a structured workout you can fit into your day to suit your circumstances, environment or the mood you are in. You
may not necessarily need to put on your exercise kit, but
it is nonetheless a time when you wedge a workout in
between other things in your day. The workout wedges
I've created have fitted into my client's days at different
times – and if they've worked for them, they can work for
you, too!

For each workout I have detailed how long they take,
how your body benefits, plus who may find this workout
particularly useful. But remember, there's no end to how
creative you can be with your workout wedges.

WALK/RUN WORKOUT WEDGE

You don't have to be Paula Radcliffe to get to grips with this mini interval training session, which combines walking and running. Interval training gets you used to working at a higher heart rate and it enables you to do more high intensity work because you get a chance to recover in between efforts. In addition, because varying the pace makes it easier for you to exercise for a longer period in total, you'll be burning lots of calories.

All levels: Warm up with 5–10 minutes walking.

Beginners: Jog for 1 minute then walk for 1 minute. Do this 5 times. Build up to 10 repetitions by adding one repetition a fortnight.

Intermediate: Jog for 1½ minutes followed by a 1½ minute walk. Do this 5 times. To progress, reduce the walking period by 10 seconds a fortnight until it equals 1 minute. Then add one extra rep per fortnight up to a maximum of 10.

Advanced: Jog for 2 minutes with a 1-minute walk in between. Repeat 5 times. Add one jog-walk repetition every fortnight until you reach a maximum of 10, then increase only your pace.

Why you should do it: It's a great calorie burner that takes minimum time.

Who should do it?: Anyone, at any life stage. As you get a little older it may well be more appropriate for you to just walk at a varying pace to have the same benefit as interval training.

How long does it take?: Between 20 and 25 minutes, depending on your level of progress.

BEACH WORKOUT WEDGE

This workout, in which the beach is your gym, is perfect for keeping yourself fit on holiday. The exercises are designed to be done on the beach without drawing too much attention to yourself. For the most part, you'll look as if you're simply enjoying your surroundings. You don't need any equipment other than what you might find on the beach (and some sunscreen, of course).

To warm up and improve aerobic fitness, start with a 20-minute walk, run or combination of the two. Running in shallow water builds aerobic fitness and strengthens the entire lower body. Pulling your feet above the surface by lifting your knees high also strengthens the abdominals. Alternatively, run on the dry sand. This is a tough one and is best kept to small bouts, as it places a lot of stress on the Achilles tendon and calf muscles if you aren't accustomed to it. Aim for five two-minute bouts. Walking on the dry sand will also burn loads of calories, or, to add variety, walk in thigh-deep water to give extra resistance.

1. Decline sit-ups

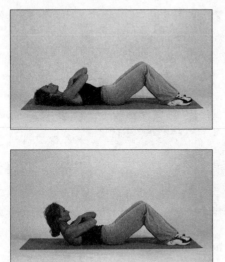

Using the decline of the beach makes these sit-ups harder than doing the exercise on a flat surface. Point your feet up the beach and your head towards the water. Bend your knees, with feet flat on the sand, hands crossed over your chest. Keeping your feet down, curl your shoulders and upper back off the sand as far as you can, keeping your belly button pulled in to your spine. Slowly lower and repeat. Do two sets of 10.

This works the abdominals.

2. Splash squat jumps

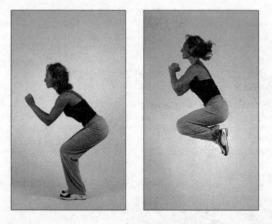

If you do these in the shallows, it'll look like you're wave jumping. Start in a squat position, legs a little wider than hip-width apart, knees bent and back straight. As the wave approaches, leap up as high as you can, landing back into the squat position. Repeat 10 times, rest then do another 10.

This works the thighs, bottom and calves.

3. Flat-out alternate lifts

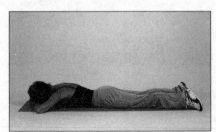

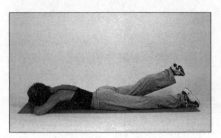

This exercise can be done lying on your beach mat or towel on a flat surface. Lie face down with forehead on the ground (or resting on your folded hands), tummy gently pulled in and legs straight and together. Pressing both hip-bones into the sand, raise the right leg by contracting the bottom and rear thigh muscles. (Think of lengthening as well as lifting the leg.) Pause and lower, then lift the left leg. Do two sets of 10 repetitions.

This works the bottom, hamstrings and lower back.

4. Wave hover

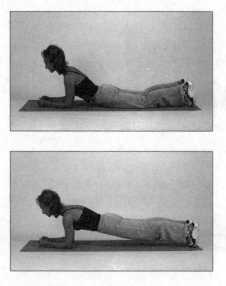

Lie face down at the water's edge as if you are cooling off, with head facing up the beach. Lift yourself up on to your elbows and forearms with your body in as straight a line as possible, keeping abdominals and glutes (buttocks) tight, feet together. Hold for the count of two waves washing up the shore then relax. Repeat 4 more times. This works the obliques (waist muscles) and the deep abdominal muscles (also known as core stabilizers) that provide stability, as well as tone, to your body. It also works the upper back and upper arms.

5. Overhead rock press

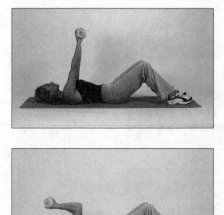

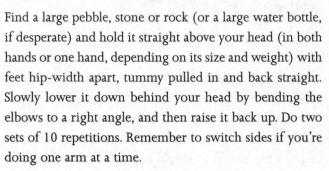

Find a large pebble, stone or rock (or a large water bottle, if desperate) and hold it straight above your head (in both hands or one hand, depending on its size and weight) with feet hip-width apart, tummy pulled in and back straight. Slowly lower it down behind your head by bending the elbows to a right angle, and then raise it back up. Do two sets of 10 repetitions. Remember to switch sides if you're doing one arm at a time.

This works the triceps at the back of the upper arms.

6. Incline push up on the rocks

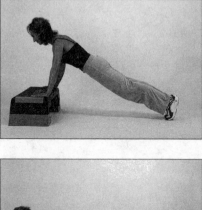

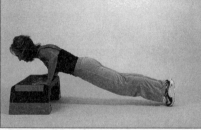

Find a rock that is about 45–60cm/18–24in high and wide enough for you to place your hands on. Put your hands on the rock, roughly shoulder-width apart with fingers pointing forward. With body straight, tummy tight and feet resting on your toes, lower your body down by bending the elbows to a right angle.

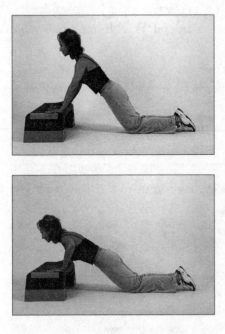

Pause then push back up. Aim for two sets of 10. If there are no rocks, use the incline of the beach by positioning yourself with your head facing up the beach, toes closest to the water. If you find this difficult, you can do the push up with your knees on the ground.

This works the chest, shoulders and upper arms.

Why you should do it: It's a great calorie burner as well as body toner – which is necessary when you consider the average person puts on around 1kg/2lb on a two-week holiday!

Who should do it?: It's especially good if you have reached your 30s, as the resistance exercise will boost your muscle mass.

How long does it take?: 30 minutes.

Tailor your gym workout to suit your needs

If you think one exercise machine is much the same as another, you're mistaken. Each one has its own special qualities and purpose – what I call their unique selling point or USP. Make the most of their differences and you can get a total body workout minus the boredom.

- Elliptical trainer's USP: easy on the joints
  Did a tough, high-impact session yesterday? The elliptical trainer is the perfect way to get a running-type workout without stressing the joints. The action is similar to running so your leg muscles will hardly know the difference and your heart and lungs will benefit, too.
- Treadmill's USP: fastest calorie burn
  If time is short and your main goal is to ramp up calorie burning, boost endurance and blast fat, jump

on the treadmill for an aerobic workout that's second to none. The treadmill is tops for guzzling the most energy.

* Exercise bike's USP: it's a no-brainer
  Tempted to give the gym a miss altogether? If your brain's frazzled and your body's fatigued, go easy by opting for the exercise bike. You don't have to worry about balance, coordination or concentration, just set the seat height, plug in your headphones and start pedalling. The mental break and gentle aerobic exercise will help you unwind and shrug off the day's stresses.

* Rowing machine's USP: upper body boost
  Most gym cardiovascular equipment focuses on the large muscles of the lower body – the butt, thighs and hamstrings. The rowing machine is different – demanding strength and endurance in the back, abdominals, arms and shoulders, as well as the legs and bum. It's a total body workout, providing you get the technique right.

* Stair climber's USP: great bum blaster
  In jumping, hopping and stepping movements the hip extensors (that's your bottom) are challenged the most – making this machine a great bottom blaster!

Fit tips

When you're on the treadmill, crank up the incline to burn 10–20 per cent more calories, whether you're walking or running. Listening to music while you exercise can make you go for longer. Upbeat music with a strong rhythm and tempo is particularly good for making people push themselves further.

PLAYGROUND WORKOUT WEDGE

Game for a laugh? This playground-inspired workout doesn't feel like exercise and it can involve all the family.

• **Leapfrog**

This uses all the body's major muscles in a propulsive manner, improving strength and power. Getting the timing right also requires good coordination.

How to play: Get your partner to stand side-on and bend, hands resting on legs or feet and head tucked in. Take a run-up, place your hands on their back and spring off the ground – taking your legs wide – and over them, landing on the other side. Now let your partner leap over you. Do 10 jumps each.

Tip: Get a good run-up or you'll land on top of them.

• **Tag**

There are lots of variations of this 'chase me' game but they have one thing in common – the aim is not to get caught!

How to play: If there are two of you, try hopping tag. Both of you can travel only by hopping and whoever is 'it' has to try to catch the other one. Once you're caught, you then become 'it'. If there's a group of you, try stuck-in-the mud. If you're caught, you stand still but another player can free you by touching your ankle. Take two-minute turns being 'it'.

Tip: If you're hopping, change legs every five to eight hops.

- **Piggyback**

Jogging or even walking with someone on your back increases the load on your cardiovascular and musculo-skeletal systems. It's good for strengthening your legs, back and abdominals.

How to play: You'll have most fun with this if you have other pairs to race. Pick a point about 30 feet/10 metres away and get on your partner's back. The piggy has to get to the finishing point as fast as possible. Jog back to the starting point and swap over. Do three runs each, rest for a minute then repeat.

Tip: For extra benefit, use your inner thighs to grip the piggy's torso.

- **Spiderman**

Even the fittest gym fan can't climb up buildings, but adopting the spiderman posture will do wonders for your abdominal strength and core stability.

How to play: Line up on the starting line on your hands and knees. When the whistle goes, crawl forward, with legs wider than hip-distance apart, tummy pulled in, bottom level with back, and hands stretched ahead of you. Move forward as quickly as possible, maintaining this position. The first person to get to the end of the room and back wins.

Tip: Use a mirror to check your body position. Your bottom should not be pointing up towards the ceiling.

• Pass the ball

This game makes you move laterally, which we rarely do in daily life, so it uses different muscle groups as well as improving agility and flexibility.

How to play: The idea is for you and a partner to carry a ball from one place to another without using your hands. You can go back-to-back with a partner, with the ball in the small of your backs, or chest-to-chest.

Tip: Communicate with your partner so that you move in unison.

• Wheelbarrows

Do you remember this? Someone holds your feet and you run along on your hands till they drop you! Well, there's a bit more technique involved in fitness wheelbarrows to make it safer and more effective.

How to play: The wheelbarrow starts in a push-up position with tummy pulled in firmly. The pusher picks up their ankles, not lifting them too high, and both walk forward, one on their hands, the other on their feet. Try to do 30 feet/10 metres, then swap over. Repeat twice.

Tip: Keep your head in line with your spine, the tummy pulled in and body in a straight line from crown to heels.

Why you should do it: As well as making you laugh as you exercise, you'll be challenging the stamina of your heart and lungs as well as your flexibility.

Who should do it?: Anyone has the ability to be a child again, but it's especially important if you are a parent as playing with your kids like this is leading by example.

How long does it take?: It's up to you but chances are it will keep the whole family entertained for at least half an hour.

EQUIPMENT-FREE WORKOUT WEDGES FOR STRENGTH

These are perfect for when the kettle is boiling, you're waiting for that return phone call or you simply need a quick break.

• Legs and bum – 5-minute blast

Do 15 repetitions of alternate rear lunges, squats and standing calf raises without a break. Rest for 30 seconds and then repeat twice more.

Alternate rear lunges

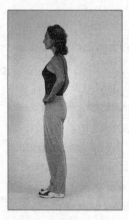 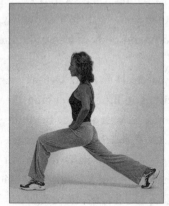

Squats

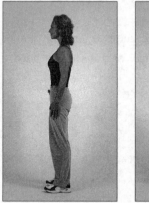 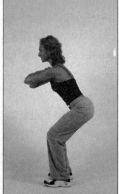

Standing Calf Raises

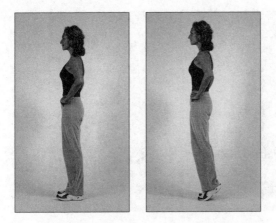

- Chest, shoulders and triceps – 2-minute toner

Do 10 counter push-ups against a kitchen counter or table, then sit on an upright chair and do 10 tricep dips.

Counter Push-ups

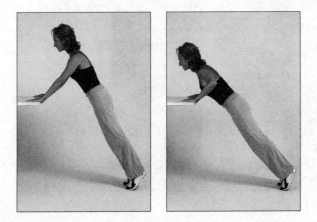

Tricep Dips

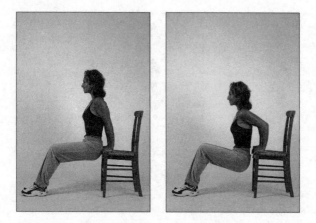

Now use a couple of cans from the store cupboard to do 10 lateral raises. Repeat the set once or twice.

Lateral Raises

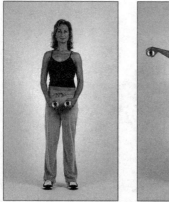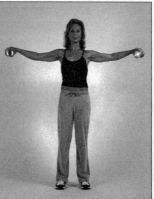

- Midriff management – 10 minutes

Try the following three tummy toners for improved muscle strength and core stability.

Alternate touchdowns: Lie on a mat with your knees bent directly over your hips and your lower legs extended at a right angle to the thighs. Contract your abdominals and pelvic floor to protect the lower back and stabilize the torso. (You should feel some tension in the abdominals maintaining this position).

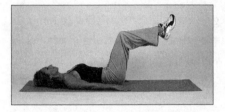

Now, slowly lower one foot forward and down to the floor, keeping the stability and control in the torso. Raise the foot back to the start position and lower the other foot. Continue alternating for the remainder of the set, breathing freely throughout. Do two sets of 12.

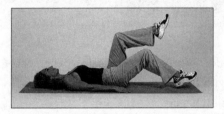

Modified T-stand: Lie on a mat on your side, with your bottom leg bent and your top leg extended with the foot on the floor. Rest your weight on your lower elbow with the forearm in front.

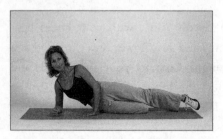

Keeping the lower leg where it is, contract your abdominals and lift your body up so that your upper leg is parallel to the floor and your weight is supported on the lower leg and elbow only. Once you feel steady, raise the upper arm directly overhead.

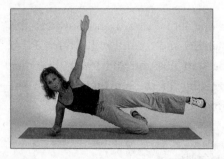

Hold for 5–15 seconds. Swap sides. As this gets easier, perform the exercise with both legs straight.

Do two reps on each side.

Crunch: Lie with your knees bent and your lower legs resting on a chair or bed – there should be a right angle at the hip and at the knee.

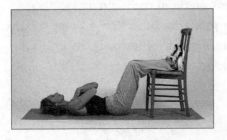

Cross your hands over your chest and curl your shoulder blades off the floor, pulling the navel to the spine and exhaling as you curl up.

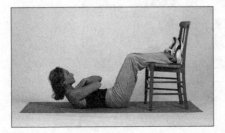

Do two sets of 10–15.

DESK WORKOUT WEDGE

This brief stretching sequence will help revive your senses, release tension and improve posture. Start by stretching your arms overhead, with interlinked fingers, and gently pushing your arms back. Now take the stretch down to the left, hold for a few seconds, return to the centre and take it down to the right.

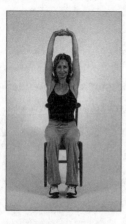 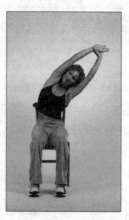

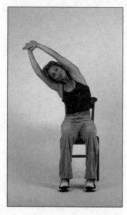

Now take hold of the back of your seat with both hands and gently lean forward, feeling a stretch near the front of your armpits. If necessary move forward in your seat until you feel a stretch.

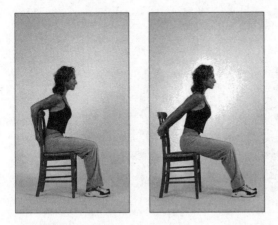

Now put interlinked fingers behind your head (elbows out to the sides). Press your head back into your hands for 5 seconds, continuing to breathe freely.

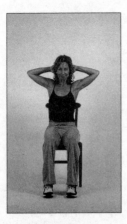

Relax and repeat 3 times. Now gently twist to your right and take hold of the back of the chair (if you can manage it, your right hand should be on left side of chair). Hold the stretch and then repeat to the left.

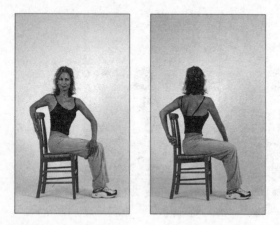

Finally, pull the chair away from the desk and lower your chest on to your thighs, allowing your arms to flop to the floor. Hold for 20 seconds.

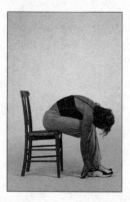

Why you should do it: As well as burning calories it's a great stress reliever.

Who should do it?: Anyone who sits down in one position for any length of time.

How long does it take?: 5 minutes.

WORKOUT WEDGE FOR GOOD BALANCE

From around the age of 40, our balance deteriorates. Tiny sensory hairs in the inner ear lose their sensitivity, decreasing our ability to detect balance changes. In addition, the mobility in our feet tends to decrease which, in turn, also affects our balance as the bones of the feet are important attachment sites for foot and leg muscles.

To improve your balance, perform the following three exercises three times a week. All you need is a chair, so you can do them at home or at the office.

• Leg back lifts

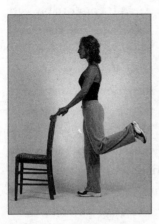

Stand with good posture, holding onto a chair. Take three seconds to slowly lift your leg back behind you, squeezing your calf close to your thigh. Hold for a second then slowly lower for three seconds. Repeat with the other leg.

• Leg front lifts

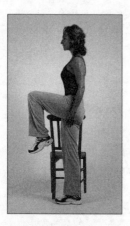

Stand sideways next to a wall or chair. Slowly raise your left knee for 3 seconds, bringing it as close as possible to your chest. Hold for 1 second and then take 3 seconds to slowly lower it. Repeat with the other leg. Make sure you stretch up through your back as you do this so the knee comes to the chest and not the chest to the knee.

• Side lifts

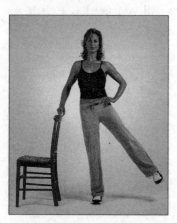

Stand sideways to a wall or chair and lift your leg out to the side, taking three seconds to take it as far as it will comfortably go. Make sure you keep your back straight as you lift. Hold for one second and then slowly lower down, taking three seconds. Repeat on the other leg. As you lift, focus on contracting your pelvic floor muscle to help your balance. The pelvic floor muscle is the one you squeeze to stop the flow of urine.

To make this exercise more challenging, try to perform it with just one finger on the wall or chair and then try it with your eyes closed. This is much harder than you may imagine, as your eyes provide an essential reference point for your brain to balance the body.

Why you should do it: Balance is important for good posture, helping you to look a size smaller. It also means you can exercise safely.

Who should do it?: Everyone will benefit but it's particularly useful for those in their late thirties and beyond. Having good balance will enhance your ability to move your body and be physically active, which means you can keep burning calories and maintain your weight and health for longer.

How long does it take?: Only 5 minutes – now that really is a small workout wedge!

The shopping workout wedge

This is so simple. How about resolving to walk twice around the shopping block or the department store before you go in? It's simple but this way you can easily build up a workout wedge of an extra 10 minutes of activity each day.

SWIM WORKOUT WEDGE

You'll tone up and burn calories with this super-effective water workout. The minimum time/max results focus of this workout means you can slot this in when taking your children for a swim, or why not add it on to a swim with your friends?

• Treading grapes

Lower body move

Take a wide stance and pump your legs up and down, lifting your knees as high as you can. Imagine you're treading grapes. Try to touch the bottom of the pool with each stride. This is a great exercise for your legs and bottom.

Upper body move

Hold your arms out in front of you, bending them slightly at the elbow. Alternatively, press each arm down hard to your hips then back up again. This works your upper back and the back and front of the arms as you bring them back up again.

• Froggie jumps

Lower body move

Take a wide stance and jump like a frog, bringing your knees to the surface and back down again, landing on the pool floor. This is great for your tummy muscles.

Upper body move

Place your hands together near the surface of the water, so they form a scoop. Reach down and then press them back up without breaking the surface of the water. You can make this harder for your waist by first pressing your arms to the left and then down to the right – this will really target your waist muscles.

- Scissor jumps

Lower body move

Stand in a lunge position with one leg in front and one behind. Now jump to swap the position of your legs, bending them as you go. This really shapes and tones your thighs, hips and bottom.

Upper body move

Stretch your arms out to the side near the surface of the water. Keep your shoulders down and back with your shoulders slightly bent. Press your arms down to the side and back up again as you change leg position. This works your shoulders and the back of your arms.

If you want to make these exercises harder use water gloves, paddles, or aquatic hand buoys for extra resistance. **Why you should do it:** Water decreases the impact on your body but it's a very effective form of resistance that tones muscles and burns calories.

Who should do it?: Anyone – though it's particularly good for new mums as the kids can play as you sneak in your workout wedge. It's also great if you're new to exercise or recovering from injury.

How long does it take?: 10 minutes.

> **Water Rules**
> 1. Exercise in navel- to chest-deep water.
> 2. Swim a couple of lengths or walk and then jog on the spot for 3 minutes as part of your warm up.
> 2. Wear water shoes to give you extra grip.
> 3. Add equipment if the exercises feel too easy.
> 4. Make sure you perform the moves well; if you increase your speed make sure it is not to the detriment of your technique.
> 5. It's a good idea to start off practising your upper and lower moves separately so you master the techniques.
> 6. Gently swim a couple of lengths to cool down.

DINNER AND A WORKOUT WEDGE

This is such a simple but effective strategy. You come home, prepare a Carb Curfew supper that takes minimum time to prepare and about 30 minutes to cook, during which time you complete a 20-minute, pre-dinner workout wedge.

I designed my dinner and workout wedge concept because I found a number of my clients enjoyed cooking, but often got tempted to snack and not exercise when they got home. Fitting a meal and some exercise into a specific time slot prevented them doing this and also meant that these things were not taking over the entire evening. Plus, of course, they also felt virtuous that they were providing a healthy meal and doing some exercise too. Piggy-backing your workout wedge with your dinner is a great way to feel good about what you are doing, it stops you wasting time and it frees up other time for you to spend with your family and friends. Many clients have also found that completing their exercise before their dinner actually helped them eat less and not pig out. It really is as simple as prep, exercise and eat!

20-MINUTE WORKOUT WEDGE IDEAS

I have chosen 20-minute workout wedges to allow you time to change into your exercise kit and get ready, but there isn't much time to hang around – so get moving! By the time you have finished your workout your Carb Curfew dinner will be ready.

Why not try …

- a 20-minute exercise video
- a walk round your neighbourhood – go for 10 minutes in one direction then turn around and come back home the same way
- the beginner's walk/run workout wedge on page 119
- the equipment-free workout wedges for strength on page 133

Here are some delicious Carb Curfew suppers that take the necessary 30 minutes to cook. They are laid out in a specific way to give you an idea of how the concept works. You'll find other recipes that work with the dinner workout wedge concept flagged up in the recipe section on pages 196–237. Once you're familiar with the idea you'll find it's quite straightforward to apply.

Thai Beef Salad
Serves 2

For the beef
2 lean beef steaks
Juice of 1 lime
1 tablespoon soy sauce

Info per serving:
Calories: 444
Fat: 19g
Protein: 36g
Carbohydrate: 25g

For the salad
150g tomatoes
100g celery
100g spring onions
100g carrot
15g coriander

For the dressing

1–2 small red chillies

1 garlic clove

1 teaspoon fish sauce

½ teaspoon palm sugar, brown sugar or honey

The prep stage:

1. Place the steaks in non-corrosive dish, pour over 2 tablespoons of the lime juice and the soy sauce and leave to one side to marinate.
2. Cut all the salad veg into strips and combine them with the coriander in a salad bowl.
3. Crush the chillies and garlic together to make a paste. Stir in 2 tablespoons of lime juice, fish sauce and sugar or honey.

Get changed and do your 20-minute workout wedge.

On returning, complete these finishing touches:

1. Heat a griddle or frying pan over a very high heat. Add the marinated steaks, turn the heat down to medium-low and cook for 1–2 minutes on each side.
2. Pour the salad dressing over the vegetables and toss well.
3. Place the vegetables on serving plates and top with the steaks.

Eat and enjoy!

Salmon, Cannellini Bean and Lemon-Infused Stew

Serves 2

225g salmon fillet, skinned and cut into
    cubes

2 lemons

½ tablespoon olive oil

1 small onion, finely chopped

1 celery stick, finely chopped

2 bay leaves

227g can tomatoes

275ml vegetable stock

Salt and pepper, to taste

227g can cannellini beans, drained

Chopped fresh parsley to garnish

Info per serving:
Calories: 314
Carbohydrate: 21g
Protein: 29g
Fat: 12g

The prep stage:

1. Grate the rind of one lemon and shred a few strips from the other. Squeeze the juice of both and set aside.

2. Heat the oil in a large pan, add the onion and celery and fry for 10 minutes.

3. Stir in bay leaves, tomatoes and stock. Season and simmer, uncovered, for 20 minutes.

Get changed and do your 20-minute workout wedge.

On returning complete these finishing touches:

1. Stir the lemon juice, grated lemon rind (keep the strips for decoration), beans and salmon into the tomato sauce and simmer for 6–8 minutes.
2. Spoon the stew into bowls and garnish with lemon strips and parsley.

Eat and enjoy!

Mexican Bean Chilli

Serves 2

75g red kidney beans
1 small red chilli
400g can chopped tomatoes
1 red pepper
1 celery stick
1 small carrot
1 garlic clove
1 teaspoon cumin
Salt and pepper, to taste
2 sprigs fresh coriander

Info per serving:
Calories: 100
Carbohydrate: 30g
Protein: 8g
Fat: 3g

The prep stage:
1. Crush the chilli to make a purée and place in a large saucepan with the canned tomatoes.
2. Chop the pepper, celery and carrot and add them to the tomatoes.
3. Crush the garlic and stir it in with the cumin.

4. Rinse and drain the beans and add them to the tomato mixture.

5. Bring the mixture to a boil, then lower the heat and simmer for 30 minutes.

Get changed and do your 20-minute workout wedge.

On returning complete these finishing touches:

1. Season to taste with salt and pepper and serve garnished with the coriander.

Eat and enjoy!

Provencal-style Poached Chicken with Vegetables

Serves 2

2 skinless, boneless chicken breasts

725ml chicken stock

4 tablespoon white wine

1 teaspoon herbes de Provence mixture

100g canned tomatoes

100g broccoli florets

100g courgettes

75g leeks

75g baby carrots

Salt and pepper, to taste

1 tablespoon finely chopped fresh parsley, to garnish

Info per serving:
Calories: 174
Carbohydrate: 20g
Protein: 32g
Fat: 4g

The prep stage:

1. Place the chicken in a frying pan with the stock, wine and herbes de Provence.
2. Bring to the boil, cover and simmer gently for about 25 minutes.
3. While the chicken is coming to the boil, cut all vegetables, except baby carrots, into bite-sized pieces and set aside.

Get changed and do your 20-minute workout wedge.

On returning complete these finishing touches:

1. Add all vegetables to the chicken and season to taste.
2. Cover and cook for another 5 minutes, or until the chicken is fully cooked and the vegetables are just tender. Sprinkle with parsley before serving.

Eat and enjoy!

THE BOTTOM LINE – WHAT YOU NEED TO DO

- Buy a pedometer – this gives an invaluable insight into how active you really are.
- Find a workout wedge appropriate to you.
- Learn to navigate your 24 hours to include lots of activity.

GET SAVVY ABOUT FATS

Most of us consider fat a dirty word when it comes to weight loss, but all fats are not created equal. Yes, fat does contain more than twice as many calories as carbohydrates or protein, but blaming fat entirely for our weight issues is misguided. People who follow a low-fat diet will not automatically shed excess pounds – in fact, I've seen many who have had just this problem. We seem to have forgotten that the body converts not just the fat we eat into body fat, but also the excess carbohydrates and protein in our diet. The combination of excess calories – regardless of where they come from – and inadequate exercise, results in the accumulation of body fat.

Many people seem to overlook this and blame their extra pounds solely on their fat intake. This is essentially why I developed my Carb Curfew concept – because more and more people were coming to me having followed low fat diets and not lost weight. What usually transpired was that although their intake of fat may well have been low, they had an excess intake of calories, particularly from carbs.

Like carbohydrates and protein, fat is an important source of energy for the body. It provides 9 calories per gram (as opposed to the 4 calories per gram provided by carbohydrates and protein) and is a particularly good source of calories for infants and young children as it supports growth and the development of tissue – about half of the calories in human breast milk, for instance, comes from fat.

Research has shown conclusively that the risk of various diseases can be lowered by reducing some types of fat in our diet, particularly the saturated fats found in animal products, full-fat dairy products, processed foods and tropical oils. Only recently has it come to light, however, that other types of fat, such as monounsaturated fats (those found in olive oil and canola oil) and omega-3 fatty acids (found in fatty fish, soy and flaxseed) can actually be beneficial to health and even fight diseases such as cancer.

MAKING FATS WORK FOR YOU

The widespread confusion surrounding fat is understandable. Some fats are described as 'healthy' others as 'bad'. Some contribute to heart disease, but others are considered 'heart-healthy'. The trick to staying healthy, and at a healthy weight, is to eat the right fats, in the right amounts (see How much fat should I be eating? on page 159). To begin to do this you first need a basic understanding of the different types of fat. Different foods contain different types and amounts of what are called fatty acids. There are three principal types of fatty acids: saturated, monounsaturated and polyunsaturated.

Saturated fatty acids are the worst of the three from a health point of view as they stimulate cholesterol production in the liver and can increase the risk of heart disease. As mentioned above, they are found mainly in dairy produce and meat, although a few oils – namely palm and coconut oil – also contain substantial amounts of saturated fatty acids.

However, although foods such as milk, yoghurt, red meat and poultry contain saturated fat, they are also excellent sources of vitamins, minerals, protein and carbohydrates so they can be consumed in moderation (though it's best to go for the low-fat options). Other foods that have a high saturated fat content – such as crisps, buttery popcorn, crackers, chips and so on – contain few beneficial nutrients and should be kept to a minimum.

In contrast to saturated fatty acids, monounsaturated and polyunsaturated fatty acids are identified as more heart-healthy. Monounsaturated fats – such as grapeseed oil, olive oil, canola oil, peanut oil, walnut oil and almond oil – can decrease liver-based cholesterol production, while polyunsaturated fats – such as corn oil, sunflower oil and cottonseed oil – are considered more or less neutral in that they don't affect it.

How much fat should I be eating?

Fat should constitute no more than 30 per cent of total calories in the diet: 10 per cent or less from saturated sources, 10 per cent or more from monounsaturated sources and about 10 per cent from polyunsaturated sources. However, that still translates into a pretty generous allowance of 50 to 60 grams of fat in a typical low-fat diet of 1,600 calories per day. In my experience, when starting out on the road to drop a size, a good rule of thumb is to aim for a total daily fat intake of no more than 40 grams. Using this as a rule of thumb gives you enough of a buffer for when you misinterpret the amount of fat in something – or for when you occasionally let your hair down.

Fats are important in the body for a number of reasons – not just because of their effect on cholesterol levels. They perform a number of essential tasks.

HOW FATS FUNCTION IN THE BODY

Fat is responsible for transporting the fat-soluble vitamins A, D, E and K. These vitamins require fat, rather than water, for absorption in the body and each is critical for maintaining optimal cell functioning. In addition, fat provides the essential oils for nails, hair and skin maintenance – so it helps prevent premature skin ageing. From a weight loss perspective, fats help to create satiety and prevent bingeing, so it's best to regard sources of healthy monounsaturated fats – for example avocado, olive oil and most nuts – as diet friendly (though of course in moderation).

There are specific types of fats that we need to perform various vital tasks within the body; these are called essential fatty acids because the body cannot produce them, they must be provided by the foods we eat.

THE ESSENTIAL FATTY ACIDS

There are two main types of essential fatty acids (EFAs); omega-3 fatty acids (linolenic acid) and omega-6 fatty acids (linoleic acid). Both are polyunsaturated fats.

Omega-3 fatty acids are found not only in oils such as flaxseed and walnut, but also in oily fish such as salmon, mackerel and sardines. Studies have shown a strong link between omega-3 fatty acid intake and reduction of triglyceride level, plasma cholesterol level and incidence of cancer (National Research Council Committee on Diet and Health 1989).

Omega-6 fatty acids are the predominant fatty acid found in vegetable oils such as soybean, corn and safflower oils. They appear to act very similarly to monounsaturated fats such as olive and canola oils. Like omega-3 fatty acids, they may protect against heart disease because of their role in producing anti-inflammatory prostaglandins.

One omega-6 fatty acid worth learning about is conjugated linoleic acid (CLA), available at the greatest levels in dairy products and beef and at lower levels in poultry, pork, fish and polyunsaturated fats. Initial research indicates that CLA has a significant role to play in cancer prevention and heart disease. It also may have a specific benefit when it comes to reducing body fat (see box page 164).

Olive oil – the best choice?

Olive oil is the principal fat in the Mediterranean diet. It is rich in monounsaturated fats, the type that lowers LDL (bad) cholesterol levels and protects HDL (good) cholesterol levels. One recent study found that people with diets high in monounsaturated fat reduced their risk of heart disease by 21 per cent, while those who simply followed a low-fat diet reduced it by only 12 per cent.

Olive oil also contributes to better control of high triglyceride levels and may reduce the risk of breast and colorectal cancers. It may also help people with inflammatory and autoimmune diseases such as rheumatoid arthritis.

How to add more olive oil to your diet:

- Stop buying store-bought salad dressings and instead mix extra virgin olive oil with your favourite vinegar.
- Use olive oil (except strongly flavoured extra virgin varieties) in place of other fats when baking.
- If serving bread with salad or a meal, place a saucer of olive oil for dipping on the table instead of the butter dish.

THE BAD GUY

Trans fats, widely discussed in the media recently, are polyunsaturated liquid oils that have been saturated with extra hydrogen atoms to make them solid. You can spot trans fats in your food by looking for the terms 'hydrogenated' or 'partially hydrogenated'. Trans fats increase the risk of cancer and heart disease and raise cholesterol levels. In fact, they may be a bigger health threat than saturated fats, as they not only raise LDL levels but also lower HDL levels, creating a double whammy as far as your heart is concerned.

Unfortunately, trans fats are a godsend to many in the food industry. The hydrogenation process lengthens the shelf life of foods, prevents rancidity and can be applied to any liquid fat. Cheese-flavoured crackers may contain partially hydrogenated soybean oil, a muesli bar may contain partially hydrogenated sunflower seed oil and cereal may contain partially hydrogenated coconut oil.

Fat categories of common foods

Foods contain more than one type of fat and hence they are categorized as a saturated, monounsaturated or polyunsaturated fat according to which type of fat is predominant. For example, margarine contains approximately 45–75 per cent polyunsaturated fatty acids, 22–50 per cent saturated fatty acids and 5–15 per cent monounsaturated fatty acids.

Consequently it could be categorized as a polyunsaturated fat. However, margarine is considered a trans fat because the oils used to make it are hydrogenated. The following table categorizes various foods in this manner.

Monounsaturated fats ('good')	Polyunsaturated fats ('good')	Saturated fats ('bad')	Trans fats ('bad')
olives	**omega-3**	coconut oil	margarine
olive oil	flaxseed oil	butter	granola bars
canola oil	salmon	beef	cookies
peanuts	mackerel	palm oil	(processed)
peanut oil	sardines	mayonnaise	snack crackers
avocados	tuna	cheese (other	pastries
avocado oil	cod liver oil	than fat-free)	(processed)
grapeseed oil	wheat germ	milk (other	chocolate
	walnuts	than fat-free)	(inexpensive)
	walnut oil	eggs	salad dressings
	peanut butter	ice cream	whipped cream
	omega-6	chocolate made	(non-dairy)
	soybean oil	with cocoa butter	some cereals
	corn oil		
	cottonseed oil		
	blackcurrant seed oil		
	safflower seed oil		

Does this tickle your G spot?

Many Hollywood dermatologists recommend a diet high in omega-3 fats, stating it plumps the skin, slows down cell degeneration and boosts the elasticity of the skin. So you may not be motivated to cut the bad fat for the sake of your health – but better looking skin may just do the trick!

Conjugated linoleic acid or CLA

While many Europeans have been steadfastly cutting out red meat and drastically limiting their intake of high-fat dairy products, all in the cause of healthier living, it turns out they may also have been depriving themselves of one of nature's important fatty acids – conjugated linoleic acid or CLA.

Studies have shown when CLA is added to the diet of rats and mice there is a decline in body fat. Swedish researchers also published promising results from a four-week study of the effects of CLA in obese men ages 39 to 64 diagnosed with metabolic syndrome X (see page ?? for more on this syndrome). Those who took the CLA supplements showed a significant decrease in abdominal fat by the end of the study.

The way in which CLA works is still to be confirmed but it is thought it increases the rate at which we burn fat, while at the same time inhibiting fat storage. However, CLA supplementation is not the golden nugget we're all looking for – yes it appears promising and it may be a useful asset in weight management but all the studies so far were particularly successful when CLA was taken in conjunction with an exercise program.

Studies suggest that health benefits are obtained from a CLA intake of around 3g a day. Certain groups of people are likely to have an even lower than average CLA intake. These include athletes on very low-fat diets and the elderly, as well as one group for whom CLA intake may be particularly important – obese people on weight-loss programs.

So what exactly is CLA?

Linoleic acid is an essential fatty acid and conjugated linoleic acid is a form of linoleic acid found in meat and dairy foods derived from ruminants – cattle, sheep and goats. Cheese, lamb, beef and beef products are among the richest food sources but for the purposes of producing natural-source dietary supplements, CLA can also be made from safflower oil rather than animal sources. CLA supplements are made by converting the linoleic acid in natural sunflower oil into conjugated linoleic acid – the same molecule as the CLA that occurs naturally in beef and dairy foods.

THE BOTTOM LINE – WHAT YOU NEED TO DO

- Eat fat every day. Our bodies use the fat we eat to produce energy, manufacture hormones such as testosterone, oestrogen and growth hormones, and absorb the fat-soluble vitamins A, D, E and K.
- Eat more foods that contain EFAs – EFAs are abundant in fish, nut oils and soybean, flaxseed, olive and canola oils. You can also take EFA supplements. Omega-3 fatty acid supplements come in the form of fish, cod liver and flaxseed oil capsules, while omega-6 supplements are sold in the form of evening primrose, borage and blackcurrant seed oil.
- Choose the healthiest fats possible. Of course, all fats increase the caloric density of food, but those laden with saturated or trans fats, such as margarine, can at least be replaced with foods rich in beneficial omega-3 and omega-6 fatty acids. After all, both a teaspoon of flaxseed oil and a teaspoon of butter or trans-fat-rich margarine contain 45 calories and 5 grams of fat, so you may as well opt for the healthier type of fat.

DON'T SKIMP ON THE PROTEIN

Protein is the essential building block for all the cells in the body. It is a component of muscle, it assists in cell maintenance and repair, it modulates insulin levels and helps regulate metabolism – and these are just some of its important roles in the body.

Protein is made up of both essential and non-essential amino acids. While non-essential amino acids can be manufactured in the body from other amino acids, the essential ones must be provided by the foods we eat. There are eight essential amino acids and all eight are present together only in foods of animal origin (for example, dairy products, fish, meat and eggs). While all the essential amino acids can be obtained from vegetable sources, none of these sources contain the full range, therefore it is necessary to combine certain foods in order to get the full quota. So for example, rice and peas are combined, or potatoes and lentils.

HOW MUCH PROTEIN DO WE NEED?

Regardless of the source, adults need 0.75g of protein per kg of body weight per day, according to the Department of Health. So if you weigh 70kg, for example, you need 52.5g of protein each day. Guidelines for active people, however, suggest that 1g may be necessary to compensate for the heavy training load, which would amount to 70g per day. A good rule of thumb is to have a serving of protein at each meal. This is especially important at lunch, when having the same visual amount of protein as starch will fuel your brain and boost your concentration in the afternoon. In practical terms, this means having something like an open chicken sandwich. You'll save yourself calories by dropping one slice of bread plus the extra proportion of protein will leave you feeling satisfied.

PROTEIN CONTENT OF SOME COMMON FOODS

Food	Protein content
1 chicken breast	42g
1 serving of lean roast beef	32g
1 salmon fillet	20g
1 serving of cod	32.5g
50g lentils	12g
50g soya beans	18g
1 matchbox size piece of Cheddar	16g
1 egg	7g
200ml glass soya milk	6g

WHY PROTEIN IS IMPORTANT IN WEIGHT LOSS

Protein contains the essential amino acid leucine. This is a muscle regulator vital to weight loss and it can be obtained only from protein sources such as beef, dairy products, poultry, fish and eggs. A recent study found that people who ate more 'high-quality' protein lost more body fat than those who ate a diet consistent with standard, high-carbohydrate dietary recommendations. It is well established that protein helps build muscle, which in turn increases our metabolic rate and activity and promotes weight loss. However, this isn't the only reason why you should eat an adequate amount of protein. Protein also creates feelings of satiety, hence you feel satisfied after a protein-rich meal. In addition, eating protein stimulates the release of dopamine in the brain (dopamine is a brain transmitter that makes us feel more alert, boosts levels of concentration and curbs lethargy).

SO SHOULD I JUST EAT PROTEIN?

No. Limiting carbohydrates may force the body to use protein and fat for fuel but, in the long run, this type of diet taxes the body because protein and fat stores that are vital for normal cellular functioning are used instead for energy. The American Heart Association (AHA) states that such diets 'aren't proven effective for long-term weight loss' and 'also pose serious health threats'. One specific health threat cited was an increased risk of kidney disorders. In addition, high protein diets discourage the consumption of fruit, vegetables and wholegrains, therefore followers miss out on vital micronutrients and disease-fighting phytochemicals. And, of course, a diet that is high in meat protein will also be high in unhealthy saturated fat. However, eating too little protein should be discouraged as a protein-deficient diet can increase the risk of certain diseases due to sub-optimal cell functioning.

THE BOTTOM LINE – WHAT YOU NEED TO DO

- Include a source of protein at each meal.
- Snack on protein-rich foods to boost feelings of alertness and satisfaction.
- Opt for more heart-healthy protein sources such as fish, lean meats and legumes.

BEWARE OF ALCOHOL –
THE HIDDEN POUND PILER

The majority of us – 90 per cent of men and 80 per cent of women – like a drink or two, so you'll be glad to hear that dropping a size for life doesn't entail giving up alcohol for life. However, there are a few points to bear in mind. Firstly, alcohol is high in calories at 7 kcal per gram of pure alcohol. Obviously drinks vary in how much pure alcohol they contain – for instance, beer contains between 3 and 6 grams per 100ml, wines have between 8 and 10 grams, while some spirits have as much as 32 grams – but it doesn't take a genius to work out how easy it is for any kind of alcohol to sabotage your weight loss plans. Secondly, alcohol cannot be used directly by the muscles – it travels straight into the bloodstream from where it has to be metabolized before the body can make use of more preferable fuel sources, such as carbohydrate or fat. It's also a diuretic, causing your body to lose water and increasing the likelihood of dehydration. Research has also shown that alcohol may be harmful to bones. A significant reduction in bone remodelling – the process of replacing old bone with new – occurs when alcohol is consumed in moderate or high amounts. However, in terms of weight management, perhaps the most significant factor is that drinking alcohol lowers your awareness of what you are eating and is likely to provoke a 'devil-may-care' attitude in which self-discipline goes out the window! One study found that just a single pre-lunch wine or beer resulted in less post-meal satiety and increased calorie intake over the next 24 hours. In other research, it has been shown that women pick poorer quality foods after even just one glass of alcohol.

Does this tickle your G spot?

Planning a workout tomorrow? Then steer clear of the booze tonight. It affects your capacity to exercise by interfering with body temperature control, dulling reflexes and perception and, of course, causing dehydration. It also delays your recovery from exercise by sapping energy levels.

ISN'T ALCOHOL MEANT TO BE GOOD FOR YOU?

As most people are now aware, there are some health benefits to be gained from drinking alcohol in *moderate* amounts. A recent study from the University of Alabama reported that moderate consumption of alcohol may decrease production and circulating levels of a clotting

protein called fibrinogen by up to 20 per cent – high
levels of fibrinogen are associated with coronary artery,
cerebrovascular and peripheral vascular diseases. Other
research associates moderate alcohol intake with a lower
risk of gallstones. Chronic heavy drinking, on the other
hand, is a leading cause of several cardiovascular illnesses,
including high blood pressure, as well as diseases of the
liver and gastrointestinal organs.

So what does 'moderate' mean? In the Alabama study
quoted above, moderate was the equivalent of two drinks
per day. So don't kid yourself that you're getting health
benefits from drinking more heavily. In addition, it has
been recognized recently that the protective effects of
alcohol on the heart are fairly modest and apply mainly to
men over 55 and women over 65.

TIPS ON A SENSIBLE ALCOHOL INTAKE

- Watch the size of your glass. Most pubs and bars serve
  wine in 175ml glasses – an official 'unit' of wine is just
  125ml, so it's easy to go overboard without realizing it.
  Half a pint of ordinary strength lager or bitter and a single
  measure of spirits constitute one unit each.
- According to Department of Health guidelines, women
  should have a maximum of 3 units per day and men 4
  units. However, their weekly guidelines are 14 units for
  women and 21 for men – so that means you can't drink
  the maximum amount of units each day!
- While it's good to have a few alcohol-free days each

week, don't 'save up' your units for the weekend.
Remember the daily guidelines and avoid binge drinking.
It overstresses the liver and is likely to lead to low energy
levels and poor eating habits.

- Mix alcoholic drinks with soft drinks or water to pace
  yourself and prevent dehydration.
- Don't eat crisps or nuts while you are drinking alcohol –
  otherwise you'll get thirstier.
- Don't drink on an empty stomach. This will slow down the
  rate at which your body can metabolize alcohol and you
  will feel drunk very quickly.
- Be extra careful if you are short, very overweight, run-
  down or tired, as your body will be less tolerant to alcohol.

THE BOTTOM LINE – WHAT YOU NEED TO DO TO DROP A SIZE

- Drink within the guidelines.
- Have two or more alcohol free days a week.
- Opt for wine or light beer rather than nutrient-deficient
  spirits.

KEEP UP YOUR WATER INTAKE

HYDRATION, HIDDEN CALORIES AND THE QUESTION OF SATIETY

All the cells of our bodies are bathed in water. It makes up 55 per cent of our blood and is essential for practically every bodily process, from energy metabolism to digestion and muscle contraction. Everyone, regardless of their activity level, needs approximately 2 litres of water a day – and if your calorie intake is significantly higher than 2000 kcals a day, then your fluid requirement is greater. If you rarely drink water and instead quench your thirst with tea, coffee or cola (which dehydrate the body), you are probably in a constant state of dehydration. Not only does this prevent your body functioning optimally, it can also hamper your weight loss efforts, as fat can only be broken down in the presence of water.

Study findings estimate that 30–40 per cent of us are mildly to moderately dehydrated. We're thought to need about 1ml of fluid per calorie of energy we consume: therefore, if your average daily intake is 1600 calories, you need a minimum of 1.6 litres of water. While a balanced diet that contains lots of fruit and veg can provide a proportion of this fluid, we should supplement these sources with drinking water itself.

SO WHAT ROLE DOES WATER PLAY IN WEIGHT LOSS?
Well, for a start, we sometimes mistake thirst for hunger, reaching for a snack when all we really needed was a drink. In addition, water helps flush out toxins and waste from the system. Perhaps of greatest importance, however, is the fact that water can have a direct impact on our energy levels – when we feel tired or lacking in energy we may reach for a sugar fix when what we need to do is rehydrate our body.

Water also swells food and helps us feel fuller – which makes us feel more satisfied. There's also evidence to suggest that foods with a high water content can help stave off hunger. Research from Penn State University found that women who were served a soup prior to their meal ate 100 less calories than those who were served a drier starter, along with a glass of water.

DRINK MORE – IT'S EASY!
The good thing about adding water to your diet is that it isn't about deprivation of anything and it doesn't take any time to do. It's simply a matter of getting used to it. Don't try to drink gallons all at once. Not only is this not an effective way for you to maintain hydration, it will also make you feel bloated and uncomfortable, especially if

you're about to do some exercise. Have a bottle of water on your desk at work, by the telephone at home and always carry a bottle in your bag.

Why it pays to stay hydrated during your workout

We lose between 500 and 1500ml of fluid per hour of exercise. A level of just 2 per cent dehydration will affect your performance, while a 4 per cent drop in hydration results in a massive 25 per cent drop in performance. Dehydration also causes a rise in heart rate, increased 'stickiness' of the blood and a far higher RPE, or perception of effort, meaning your exercise feels harder. It also dulls mental function. Follow these guidelines to ensure you avoid dehydration when you work out.

Before: Consume 300ml to half a litre of fluid 15 to 30 minutes before your workout.

During: Aim to drink 125–250ml every 15 minutes during your workout. Don't wait until you're thirsty – thirst is the body's last response to dehydration. You don't need a sports drink unless you are exercising for an hour or more – water will do just fine.

After: Following a particularly long or tough session, you may want to rehydrate with a sports drink, or a carbohydrate-rich fluid such as orange juice or fruit-flavoured squash. Drink at least half a litre of fluid after your cool down exercises and keep drinking regularly for the next few hours until your urine is the colour of pale straw or lighter.

Tip

Experts believe that water is best absorbed when drunk at room temperature rather than icy cold. The number one reason people fail to drink enough water is the taste – or lack of taste. Add a squeeze of lime or lemon, or infuse a slice of fresh ginger, if you think water tastes too dull on its own.

THE BOTTOM LINE – WHAT YOU NEED TO DO

- Aim to drink 2 litres of fluid a day; it doesn't have to be plain water but remember it is calorie free.
- Consume more liquid-based foods such as soups, smoothies and stews, to increase satiety.
- Go easy on diuretic drinks such as tea and coffee, caffeinated soft drinks and alcohol.
- Eat plenty of water-packed veg and fruit.

GET TO GRIPS WITH
PORTION CONTROL

You may not have noticed, but the packet and portions sizes of the foods we buy are getting bigger beneath our very noses. You may still be having your one muffin or bagel, but the fact is serving sizes are now two to five times larger than they were when such foods were first introduced into our supermarkets.

Even a chocolate bar has grown more than 10 times since they were first introduced. So despite the fact that you may be having just 'one', that one may now be big enough for three! And larger portions mean more calories – there's simply no getting away from it.

Thanks to supersized portions, it's estimated that we are eating 150 calories per day more than we were 20 years ago. That adds up to an extra 15 pounds per person per year. Learning to downsize is one way to prevent your waistline from expanding. Whatever way you look at it, portion control goes hand in hand with weight control. However, knowing exactly what is a portion can be a challenge – the following chart will help you size up your servings.

Food	What a serving should look like
Peanut butter (1 tablespoon) 16g fat/190 calories	size of a jaffa cake
Dry spaghetti (50g/2oz) 1g fat/211 calories	the diameter of a 10p piece
Bagel (1 small) 1g fat/190 calories	size of a 150g can of tuna
One muffin (bran) 5g fat/179 calories	size of a tennis ball
Mashed potatoes (½ cup) 9g fat/112 calories	half a cricket ball
Swiss cheese (30g/1oz) 8g fat/107 calories	pair of dice
Meat, chicken, fish (100g/4oz) 7.5g fat/165 calories (average)	a deck of cards
Low-fat vanilla ice cream (½ cup) 3g fat/92 calories	half of an orange
Dry-roasted peanuts 28g 14g fat/166 calories	one and a half golf balls
Low-fat muesli (½ cup) 3g fat/186 calories	a fist
Crisps 28g 10g fat/152 calories	half of a grapefruit

Does this tickle your G spot?

Many studies report the benefits of restricting calories and even suggest that doing so may increase your life expectancy. Watching your portion size is one simple way to do this.

Check the number of servings

This may sound obvious but how many times do you buy a ready-prepared meal, eat it and then discover it was actually designed to serve two. Read your labels carefully as sometimes the calories that are flagged up on the front of the pack relate to a 100g serving or half a pack – not the whole amount!

THE BOTTOM LINE – WHAT YOU NEED TO DO

- Read your labels to find out exactly what a portion is and try to stick to that portion size.
- Familiarize yourself with what a portion should look like. See the table opposite.
- Ditch the trendy white oversized dinner plate and get a more realistic-sized plate that won't look half empty with a normal-sized meal on it.

FOLLOW THE 80-20 RULE

Not having to be good 100 per cent of the time is vital to losing weight and keeping it off. For this reason I encourage people to follow my 80-20 rule, which basically means that if you can apply my 10 'fundamentals' 80 per cent of the time you will lose weight and keep it off. We can't be angels 100 per cent of the time – life just doesn't allow us to be and life is about having a good time and enjoying your food and exercise. If we fool ourselves that we can always be good it simply leads to disappointment and the classic dieter's get-out clause – 'well, I've blown it now so I might as well give up!'

In my experience this fundamental is enormously reassuring for my clients, particularly once they have dropped a size. Many have lost weight before only to regain it and more. These 'rebound' pounds can in part be explained by them not being in the right space to keep that size off (if this relates to you, turn back to section one to remind yourself of the skills you learnt earlier) but it is also because their weight loss was based on an unrealistic diet plan that was never going to fit in with their post-diet life. It was the classic one-night-stand diet – it gave that quick fix, but it was never going to last!

Of the 10 fundamentals some will be easier for you to master than others, but you don't need to put them into practice 100 per cent of the time to reap rewards. Of all the fundamentals, the one I would most encourage you to master is my Carb Curfew.

Case Study: Jane's Success

'I found this plan so simple and therefore easy to stick to. The only thing that I have permanently stuck to is the carbs rule and I have seen results that I am really pleased with. I still drink wine almost every day, go to restaurants and exercise in a limited way but I have nevertheless achieved weight loss not previously experienced.' Jane lost 6.3kg/1st and dropped two sizes.

Everyone wants to know how long it is going to take to drop a size and obviously the more closely you follow the plans I have devised and the fundamentals, the quicker you will experience the results. However, we are all different and if you have a dieting history you may find it takes you longer to drop a size than a friend who is following the same plan. This is not uncommon and I have seen it in a number of clients who have experienced plateaus in their weight loss, despite feeling they are putting all the fundamentals into practice. Vivian's situation is a prime example.

Case Study: Vivian's Story

Vivian was a magistrate. She had always been a wonderful, larger-than-life character who had routinely tried to lose weight but would lose a little and then gain it all back. She loved life and life loved her, however, her size, with a BMI of 29, was not going to help her enjoy the type of life she loved for as long as she would like. Vivian joined my 10-week weight management course and after seven weeks of following the eating plans, and doing plenty of exercise, she had only lost two pounds. She felt better and had more energy but she was frustrated that her efforts were not really being rewarded on the scales – and she made it very clear to me too!

I encouraged her to have patience and stick with it and explained that her body needed to continue to receive the right foods in the right quantities so that she was giving it a consistent message. The delay in her seeing and feeling the drop in size was her body's way of adjusting to what it was being asked to do. It had received so many confusing signals in the past that it needed consistency before it was able to 'trust' what was being asked of it. Just three weeks later Vivian had dropped 13 pounds! She was thrilled. What's more, four years down the line she has gone on to lose a further stone, she looks 10 years younger and has experienced no rebound pounds!

I know it can be so frustrating to be in a stalemate situation where your body isn't losing weight or changing size. One of the simplest ways I can illustrate why this happens is to get you to think about your cells, those micro biological cells that make up the human body. When we want to change our size we need to give our cells a consistent message. For our body to get smaller we need to develop a relationship with our cells, so our cells trust us and work effectively for us – we need to build and nurture a relationship with our cells. If we are constantly trying lots of different one-night-stand diets, then our cells get confused about what exactly we want them to do. Insufficient calories followed by excess calories and excessive amounts of certain food groups can really mess up our cells – they get confused and, in response, insulin levels and blood glucose levels surge and fall as the cells try to deal with the rocky road we've sent them on.

When you follow the Drop a Size for Life plan you may experience a plateau in your weight loss but rather than looking at this negatively, think about it positively. If you are following the fundamentals and operating the 80-20 rule you are developing a great relationship with your cells. They will learn to trust you and you'll drop that size and keep it off without having to put your life on hold. The great news is the longer you apply the fundamentals, the better and more trusting a relationship you develop with your cells. You'll find you start to sail through holidays, Christmas and other occasions without the significant gain in weight experienced in the past.

Case Study: Judith's Story

'I have been following Joanna's plan for five years now. The first year I started was just before Christmas. I was the classic yo-yo dieter. I wanted to drop a size for Christmas before gaining it all again over the festivities as I normally did. Well I lost the weight and dropped two sizes but come January 4, I had gained nine pounds back. I got back on track and over the next 12 months really worked at making the fundamentals part of my life. I can assure you I was not fanatical – I run a business and have three teenage kids so life is full on. Come the following Christmas, I had managed to stay at my new size all year – despite holidays and family traumas – but I knew Christmas was the real test. I like to enjoy myself at this time, and that includes my food and drink! So, come January, I was delighted to see I had only gained three pounds. Every Christmas since, I have gained weight – but not the normal 9–10 pounds I had done in the past, more like two to three. I get back on track, focus especially hard on the Carb Curfew and portion sizes and I'm soon back to that smaller size again.'

The 80-20 rule isn't an excuse for a weekend blow-out

It's false economy to try to be extra vigilant during the week, cutting your calories to a bare minimum Monday through to Friday, only to overindulge Friday night through to Monday morning. Even though this may sound like you're being 'good' 5 days out of 7, this will not help your long-term efforts to drop a size. Asking your cells to survive on very few calories for five days and then sub-jecting them to a calorie and nutrient overload for two days will hinder the relationship you are nurturing with your cells. Remember, you need to provide a consistent message, so huge variations in calories and nutrients are not good news.

If you know you are going to a party at the weekend or you enjoy feeling more relaxed about your eating habits on Saturday and Sunday, then it's better to eat a little less Monday through Friday rather than go all out on starva-tion mode. Enjoy the weekend but don't go too mad, even if you are planning to get back on track on Monday with a cardio workout wedge! This way you will be encourag-ing your cells to trust you and they'll reward you by help-ing you drop that size.

THE DROP A SIZE
EATING PLANS

Now you know the fundamentals, you can put them into practice for yourself. However, if you would like a little more guidance you can follow the simple, easy-to-follow eating plans featured in this section. To drop a size and then keep it off you need to put the fundamentals into practice right through the year. And because your taste buds, food choices and cooking methods change during the year, I've devised simple summer and winter eating plans that reflect the availability of foods and what you may prefer to eat at these different times of the year. Most people think of salads when they need to lose weight, but a cold salad may be the last thing you feel like when it's freezing outside. Conversely, a healthy veggie soup may be a great low-calorie lunch but you just may not fancy a bowl of piping hot soup when it's 25 degrees outside.

Choosing foods that you really don't want to eat can leave you unsatisfied, which in turn makes it harder to resist the biscuit tin or the toast! We all have things we like and dislike, so the plans are just guides to get you on the road. They're easy to follow – all you need to do is select a breakfast, lunch and Carb Curfew dinner option, plus one or two snacks (depending on how much you've eaten at mealtimes). You'll find a list of the options below; the recipes follow on pages 196–231 (note that not all the suggestions require recipes).

Remember the following each day:
- drink 2 litres of water spread throughout the day
- eat at least 6 servings of fruit and veg a day
- avoid going for too long without eating
- operate my Carb Curfew.

❧ WINTER EATING PLAN

BREAKFASTS

High-fibre cereal with semi-skimmed milk and ½ a banana

Poached egg on 1 slice wholemeal toast with glass of fruit juice

Bacon Sandwich and juice

Warm Fruit Compote

Veggie Breakfast

Protein-powered Porridge with Pear

Hot Milk Breakfast Shake

LUNCHES

Jacket Potato with Beans and Cheese

Chunky Vegetable Soup with Chicken

Ham and Mushroom Omelette

Toasted Sweet Chicken and Chutney Sandwich

Lentil and Sweet Potato Soup

Three-coloured Tortilla Wrap

CARB CURFEW DINNERS

One-pan Chicken

Runner Bean and Mushroom Bake

Gammon and Two-coloured Cabbage Fry

Lamb Steaks with Roasted Beetroot

Thai Salmon with Wilted Hot Vegetable Salad

Chunky Haddock Chowder with Spring Onions and
   Sweetcorn

Quick Vegetarian Chilli

SNACKS

Choose one 100-calorie snack and one 150-calorie snack
from those listed on page 194.

ᴄᵇᴑ SUMMER EATING PLAN

BREAKFASTS

Pineapple Carrot Smoothie

Wholemeal Toast with Cottage Cheese and Tasty Toms

Melon, Cheese and Crispbread
Berry Berry Crunchy Yoghurt
Boiled Egg and Toast with Virgin Bloody Mary

LUNCHES

Houmous and Salad Pitta Pocket
Open Nutty Chicken and Watercress Sandwich
Speedy Chilled Pea Soup with Savoury Cottage Cheese
Italian Stallion Bean and Tuna Salad
Speedy Gazpacho with a Tasty Topping
Prawn-stuffed Cucumber Boats

CARB CURFEW DINNERS

Easy Beef Moussaka
Ratatouille Tuna Supper
Aromatic Summer Salmon with Grape and Chilli Mango
  Salsa
Chicken and Aubergine Supper
Home-made Burgers with Tomato and Cucumber Salad
Prawn and Watermelon Salad
Middle Eastern Chicken Salad with Tahini Dressing

SNACKS

Choose one 100-calorie snack and one 150-calorie snack
from those listed on page 194.

⮑⮑ SNACKS

Snacking is an important part of the Drop a Size for Life plan, as it helps stabilize your blood glucose levels throughout the day and stops you reaching the end of the day feeling exhausted and as if you could eat a horse! Generally speaking, a snack is anything consumed outside of your regular mealtimes. However, using that criteria, a chocolate bar and a can of coke can be viewed as a snack – but they're not the kind that will power you through the day and give you a health boost, all without piling on the calories! As well as avoiding sweet snacks you should steer clear of processed snacks as much as possible, as the sodium content is usually high and the nutrient content low. Applying the following criteria to your choice of snacks will help ensure they provide energy and stave off hunger, as well as contributing to your weight loss efforts. Try to choose a snack that provides …

1. Some fluid to hydrate you.
2. A source of protein to make you feel more alert.
3. Some fat to give a feeling of fullness.
4. A source of fruit or vegetables.

Of course, not all your snacks will fulfil all the criteria but these four points are a good ideal to aim for. Here are some snack ideas that fall within different calorie brackets, so you can pick and choose depending on how hungry you are and what else you have eaten during the day.

100-CALORIE SNACKS

½ an apple spread with a teaspoon of peanut butter, plus a
glass of water

Small glass of skimmed milk

15 walnut halves with a small glass of diluted OJ

Cup of miso soup and 4 crab sticks

Chilled chocolate shake – dissolve a sachet of low calorie
instant hot chocolate mix, top up with 100ml cold water
and 100ml skimmed milk. Blend with ice for your instant
chocolate smoothie

1 rice cake with a thin spreading of ripe avocado and a slice
of lean ham or smoked salmon, plus a glass of water

10 cashew nuts and a kiwi fruit

150-CALORIE SNACKS

200ml carrot juice with a low-fat digestive biscuit and a
slither of Cheddar cheese

10g chocolate and a large glass of skimmed milk

20g dried raisins and nuts and a mini pro biotic yoghurt drink

Small can pink salmon, half a cucumber and a glass of water

2 crispbreads with cottage cheese topped with teaspoon of
Thai sweet chilli sauce

1 Matzos cracker with 2 slices thin ham, plus a small glass of
mango juice

Fruit shake – a low-fat fruit yoghurt blended with a handful
of strawberries, some ice cubes and 100ml skimmed milk

Eating out at lunchtime

Obviously, it won't always be possible to make your own lunch so you can also buy any shop-bought sandwich, sushi or salad that has less than 350 calories. Ideally, if eating shop-bought sandwiches, ditch one slice of bread to help cut the calories and boost your protein intake with a low-fat yoghurt for dessert.

If you have one near you, a soup shop is a great place to find a healthy lunch option. Select a non-creamy, vegetable-based soup that has some source of protein, such as a chicken and vegetable broth. If the calorie breakdown is listed, select one containing less than 40 calories per 100ml – but you can go for the largest serving size! If you're a vegetarian, add protein in the form of a handful of nuts (see page 242 for ideas on how to pack in the nuts without overloading on the calories).

A few words about bread

Bread is a great British dietary staple and while it can provide a range of nutrients, it's important to choose wisely. White processed bread has the greatest impact on your blood glucose levels and has the least nutrients (it may have 'added' nutrients but these are difficult for the body to assimilate), so always choose wholemeal options.

Bread is also a great culprit of supersizing! A single slice of bread can vary enormously between brands and types – so, as always, read the label. You don't have to choose diet bread, but I do urge you to select smaller loaves and less thick slices. There can be a 50-calorie difference between one brand and another.

THE RECIPES

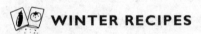 **WINTER RECIPES**

BREAKFASTS

Bacon Sandwich
Serves I

Grill three rashers (100g) of lean bacon and sandwich between two small slices of wholemeal toast. Serve with a glass (200ml) of fruit juice.

Info per serving:
Calories: 346
Carbohydrate: 43g
Protein: 25g
Fat: 9g

Warm Fruit Compote
Serves 2

50g mixed dried fruit

1 orange

100g fresh or canned pineapple

5 almonds

1 tablespoon pumpkin seeds

1 teaspoon linseeds

1 teaspoon mixed spice

125ml orange juice

150g low-fat natural yoghurt

> **Info per serving:**
> Calories: 210
> Carbohydrate: 45g
> Protein: 4g
> Fat: 4g

Put all the ingredients, except the yoghurt, in a saucepan on a low heat, cover and simmer for about 20 minutes. Serve with the yoghurt.

Veggie Breakfast
Serves 1

1 tablespoon olive oil

1 bunch spring onions, chopped

25g cherry tomatoes, halved

125g sliced mushrooms

1 pinch mixed herbs

50g silken firm tofu, cut into cubes

1 slice wholemeal bread

> **Info per serving:**
> Calories: 230
> Carbohydrate: 17g
> Protein: 9g
> Fat: 16g

Heat the oil and when it is very hot, add all the vegetables, herbs and tofu and stir-fry quickly for 3–4 minutes. Pile the mixture onto the bread and season with pepper.

Serve with a glass of milk.

Protein-powered Porridge with Pear

If you suffer from mid-morning hunger pangs, this is the breakfast for you. The oats, with their low glycaemic load, will stabilize your blood glucose all morning, while the protein powder will help make it extra filling.

Serves 1

40g porridge oats
1 small pear
20g protein powder

Info per serving:
Calories: 327
Carbohydrate: 46g
Protein: 25g
Fat: 6g

Place the oats in a pan with 1 cup of water and bring to the boil. Chop the pear and add to the porridge. Gently simmer for 2 minutes. Just before serving, stir in the protein powder.

Hot Milk Breakfast Shake

This quick and easy recipe is rich in fibre and the taste of the chocolate is really satisfying.

Serves 1

280ml skimmed milk

50g canned pitted prunes in natural juice

Sachet of low-cal hot chocolate dissolved
    in a little water

2 tablespoons wheatgerm

> **Info per serving:**
> Calories: 197
> Carbohydrate: 33g
> Protein: 12g
> Fat: 2g

Put all the ingredients in a blender and blend for 30 seconds. Transfer to a microwave container and heat through until hot. Drink straightaway or pour into a flask and enjoy later on.

LUNCHES

Jacket Potato with Beans and Cheese

Serves 1

1 small jacket potato

2 tablespoons baked beans

1 tablespoon grated Edam cheese

2 teaspoons Benecol margarine

> **Info per serving:**
> Calories: 458
> Carbohydrate: 83g
> Protein: 24g
> Fat: 3g

Bake the potato either in the oven or microwave. When the potato is almost ready, warm the baked beans. Split the potato open, fill with the Benecol and top with the warmed baked beans and the grated cheese. Put under a hot grill to melt the cheese.

Chunky Vegetable Soup with Chicken
Serves 2

600ml any fresh vegetable soup less than
    40 calories per 100g
100g roast chicken or any other leftover
    lean meat, chopped
50g frozen peas

> **Info per serving:**
> Calories: 190
> Carbohydrate: 13g
> Protein: 24g
> Fat: 4g

Warm through the soup, add the chopped chicken and continue to heat until the chicken is warmed through. Add the frozen peas and continue to heat until the peas are thawed and hot.

This sort of soup is good served with a slice of marmite toast.

Note: If buying ready-cooked chicken, choose plain, poached or chargrilled rather than the smoked or flavoured meat. You'll save yourself quite a lot of salt.

Ham and Mushroom Omelette
Serves 1

3 eggs (use all 3 egg whites but only 2 of the yolks)
A small pinch of salt and freshly ground pepper
100g chopped unsmoked lean ham (or substitute with cubed
    tofu)
1 small cooked potato, cubed

1 teaspoon olive oil
50g chopped mushrooms or any other
   leftover cooked vegetables

Info per serving:
Calories: 258
Carbohydrate: 9g
Protein: 19g
Fat: 16g

Whisk the egg whites until fairly stiff then fold in the two egg yolks and season lightly. Gently fold in the chopped ham and cooked potato. Heat a small non-stick omelette pan and add the olive oil. Pour in the egg mixture and add the mushrooms or leftover veg. Gently lift the edges of the omelette and move into the centre of the pan so all the egg mixture sets and the bottom starts to turn golden brown. Some people like their eggs very set, I prefer mine slightly on the soft side. When the eggs are done to your liking, fold the omelette over and serve.

Toasted Sweet Chicken and Chutney Sandwich
Serves 1

Info per serving:
Calories: 338
Carbohydrate: 32g
Protein: 25g
Fat: 8g

2 slices thin wholemeal bread
1 teaspoon Benecol margarine
25g mango chutney
25g low-fat cottage cheese
2 slices lean unsmoked chicken or any
   leftover roast chicken
1 medium tomato, sliced

Spread one side of each slice of bread with the margarine. Place one slice, margarine side down, on a sandwich toaster and layer on the mango chutney, cottage cheese, sliced chicken and tomato then top with the second piece of bread, margarine side up. Close the toaster and toast until your sandwich is golden brown. Generally this takes 2 minutes but will vary depending on the make of toaster.

If you don't have a sandwich toaster you can create the same effect by simply putting your sandwich in a heated non-stick pan; press it down with a large flat spatula as it cooks and once it's golden brown, turn it over to cook the other side.

Lentil and Sweet Potato Soup
Serves 2

1 small red onion, finely chopped

1 garlic clove

1 teaspoon olive oil for frying

500ml vegetable stock

1 large sweet potato, peeled and diced

120g can green lentils, drained

1 teaspoon cumin

Info per serving:
Calories: 234
Carbohydrate: 36g
Protein: 8g
Fat: 8g

Fry the onion and garlic in the olive oil until the onion is soft and browning. Pour the vegetable stock into a saucepan and add the sweet potato, lentils, onion and garlic mixture and the cumin. Simmer for 45 minutes with the lid on (perfect opportunity for a lunchtime workout wedge). Purée half the soup in a blender, mix it back into the saucepan and serve.

Three-coloured Tortilla Wrap
This recipe is also suitable for the summer months – simply substitute ½ a small ripe avocado for the cream cheese.

Serves 1

1 large (23cm) flour tortilla
1 tablespoon low-fat cream cheese
Handful of spinach leaves
2 slices smoked salmon
Packet of miso soup

Info per serving:
Calories: 303
Carbohydrate: 41g
Protein: 19g
Fat: 7g

Lay the tortilla flat and spread with the cream cheese. Next layer on the spinach leaves, covering the tortilla until you can't see any of the cream cheese. Next, lay the salmon over the spinach, covering as much of the spinach as possible. Roll the tortilla into a long fat cigar shape, cut in two on the diagonal and serve with a bowl of hot miso soup.

CARB CURFEW DINNERS

One-pan Chicken
Serves 2

1 tablespoon olive oil

2 skinless, boneless chicken breasts

1 large garlic clove

1 tablespoon honey

1 teaspoon soy sauce

125g sliced mushrooms

225g bag baby spinach

1 tablespoon pine nuts

Info per serving:
Calories: 302
Carbohydrate: 17g
Protein: 32g
Fat: 13g

Heat the oil in a non-stick wok or large frying pan. Cut the chicken into bite-size pieces and add to the pan along with the garlic, honey, soy sauce and mushrooms; fry for 5–8 minutes, keeping the pieces moving all the time to avoid sticking and to ensure the chicken is thoroughly cooked. Now add the spinach and pine nuts, cover the pan and allow to steam for a further 5 minutes before serving.

Runner Bean and Courgette Bake

This is a meal in itself but it also works well as a tasty accompaniment to cold roast meats.

Serves 2

4 large eggs

Pinch of salt and pepper

140ml skimmed milk

350g lightly steamed runner beans

200g finely sliced courgettes

1 red pepper

200g bag ready-to-cook spinach

5 walnuts, chopped

1 teaspoon olive oil

25ml lemon juice

Info per serving:
Calories: 323
Carbohydrate: 12g
Protein: 26g
Fat: 18g

Preheat the oven to 180°C/350°F/Gas mark 5.

Lightly steam the runner beans for about 4 minutes so they are **'al dente'**. Add the sliced courgettes and cook for a further minute. Meanwhile, beat the eggs with the seasoning and leave to one side. Drain the vegetables and add to the mix so all the ingredients are covered. Pour into a medium-sized ovenproof dish. Place in the middle of the oven and cook for 20 minutes or until the eggs are set. Steam the spinach, drain, squeeze a little lemon juice over it, drizzle with the olive oil and add the chopped walnuts. Toss and serve alongside the bean bake.

Semi or skimmed milk?

I am always being asked if it is necessary to switch from semi-skimmed milk to skimmed milk. Well in my opinion, this isn't vital – what is important is that you don't use full-fat milk. You can switch to skimmed if you wish, but if you really don't like the taste of skimmed then use semi. When you're cooking it's much easier to disguise the taste, so I would advise using skimmed in this situation. The difference in calories between a glass of semi-skimmed milk and skimmed milk is very small, so as long as you're not drinking too much of it – it is after all a source of saturated fat – I suggest you drink the one you prefer.

Gammon and Two-coloured Cabbage Fry
Serves 2

1 tablespoon olive oil
1 large onion, chopped
½ head red cabbage, shredded
1 teaspoon garlic paste
½ head savoy cabbage, shredded
1 large gammon steak (about 200g),
   naturally cured

Info per serving:
Calories: 309
Carbohydrate: 8g
Protein: 30g
Fat: 16g

Heat the olive oil in a large pan, add the chopped onion, red cabbage and garlic paste, stir and cover with a well-fitting lid. Turn the heat to very low and stir every 5 minutes or so as the red cabbage and onion starts to soften and sweat. After 10 minutes, add the savoy cabbage and cover. Continue to cook the two cabbages, keeping the heat low, for a further 15 minutes, stirring every 5 minutes or so. Meanwhile, cube the gammon and add to the cabbage; continue to cook until the vegetables and gammon are cooked through and the cabbage is soft and sweet.

Lamb Steaks with Roasted Beetroot

Serves 2

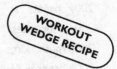

6 small whole beetroot, peeled

1 tablespoon olive oil

100ml orange juice

½ teaspoon garlic paste

2 lamb steaks with the fat cut off

2 small sprigs rosemary

90g frozen mixed vegetables

Info per serving:
Calories: 236
Carbohydrate: 11g
Protein: 30g
Fat: 7g

Preheat the oven to 200°C/400°F/Gas mark 6.

Place the beetroot in a roasting dish and pour over the olive oil and orange juice. Cover with a large sheet of aluminium foil and roast for 50 minutes. Meanwhile, rub the garlic paste over the lamb steaks, sprinkle with the rosemary and leave to one side. About 5 minutes before serving, put the grill on high and grill the lamb steaks until just pink. Steam the vegetables and serve with the roasted beetroot and lamb.

You can swap the lamb for any other meat – I've made this with beef steaks and they have gone down really well.

Thai Salmon with Wilted Hot Vegetable Salad
Serves 2

150g bag rocket or spinach salad

1 vegetable stock cube (reduced salt)

200g shallots

200g courgettes

200g mushrooms

200g broccoli florets

2 salmon fillets (about 200g), preferably organic

2 tablespoons Thai sweet chilli sauce

1 tablespoon olive oil

1 tablespoon balsamic vinegar

Info per serving:
Calories: 364
Carbohydrate: 31g
Protein: 32g
Fat: 15g

Place the rocket or salad leaves in a large bowl and leave to one side.

Dissolve the stock cube according to the pack instructions, place the stock in a large saucepan and bring to the boil. Add the shallot and simmer for about 3 minutes until they are just tender. Meanwhile, roughly chop the courgettes and mushrooms. I like the mushrooms to be quite chunky so if using button mushrooms keep them whole. Just as the shallots are starting to turn tender, add the courgettes, mushrooms and broccoli and cook for a further

2 minutes. The vegetables will still be slightly under-cooked but that's okay as they will continue cooking in the residual heat. Drain the veg and leave to one side with the lid on.

Heat the grill and place the two salmon fillets on a piece of foil, skin-side up. Grill the fish until the skin just starts to blister, turn over and grill until golden on the other side. In the meantime, heat a small non-stick frying pan and add the Thai sweet chilli sauce. Add the cooked veg and toss the veg to pick up the flavour of the sauce.

Whisk the oil and vinegar together and drizzle the mixture around the sides of the salad bowl. Quickly toss the veg through the salad, so the heat of the veg starts to wilt the salad greens. Place the salad and veg in the salad bowl and toss. Place the grilled salmon on top and serve.

Chunky Haddock Chowder with Spring Onion and Sweetcorn

Serves 2

1 head of fennel, trimmed
600ml carton fresh chilled haddock
    chowder
165g can sweetcorn (drained weight)
100g spring onions, chopped
140ml skimmed milk

Info per serving:
Calories: 252
Carbohydrate: 36g
Protein: 14g
Fat: 7g

Roughly chop the fennel and cook in a pan of boiling water for about 5 minutes. Drain and set aside. In the same pan, gently heat the chowder then add the sweetcorn, spring onions, milk and fennel. Heat through and serve in warmed bowls.

Quick Vegetarian Chilli
Serves 4

1 tablespoon olive oil

1 large onion, finely chopped

1 garlic clove, crushed

2 fresh green chillies, seeded and finely chopped (or ½–1 teaspoon chilli powder)

2 red peppers, chopped

2 carrots, diced

425g can red kidney beans, drained

400g can chopped tomatoes

2 courgettes, diced

125g low-fat natural yoghurt

Info per serving:
Calories: 192
Carbohydrate: 33g
Protein: 8g
Fat: 4g

Heat the oil in a large saucepan and fry the onions in it. Add the garlic and chilli when the onions begin to soften and cook for a few minutes, stirring. (Add a little water if the oil dries up). Now add all the remaining ingredients, except the courgettes and yoghurt, stir well, cover and cook over medium heat for 15 minutes. Add the courgettes, and simmer for a further 5 minutes, or until all the vegetables are cooked through. Serve with a dollop of the yoghurt.

Tip

This recipe freezes well, so make double and freeze it in individual portions for a convenient meal for one.

Fresh garlic and garlic purée

Garlic purée is available from most supermarkets and is a great standby for when you are really short of time. When using fresh garlic – which, if time allows, I definitely prefer – peel and chop it, then let it rest for 10–15 minutes before you heat it. Heating right away does not allow time for the heart-protecting, cancer-fighting compounds, called allicins, to be activated.

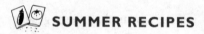 **SUMMER RECIPES**

BREAKFASTS

Pineapple Carrot Smoothie

This may sound like an odd mixture but it's delicious and super healthy. The carrot purée provides an easily absorbable form of beta-carotene, which studies suggest cuts the risk of breast and possibly ovarian cancer.

Serves I

1 pot baby food carrot purée, chilled
150ml pineapple juice, chilled
Ice cubes

Info per serving:
Calories: 122
Carbohydrate: 31g
Protein: 1g
Fat: 1g

In a blender, blend the carrot purée, pineapple juice and ice. Pour into a glass and drink straightaway.

Wholemeal Toast with Cottage Cheese and Tasty Toms

Serves I

6 cherry tomatoes
½ tablespoon olive oil
Pinch of mixed herbs
1 slice wholemeal toast
100g low-fat cottage cheese

Info per serving:
Calories: 162
Carbohydrate: 21g
Protein: 16g
Fat: 3g

Heat the grill, slice the cherry tomatoes in half and place on the grill pan, face up. Drizzle with the olive oil and sprinkle on the herbs. Grill until the tomatoes just begin to bubble. Meanwhile, spread the wholemeal toast with the cottage cheese and, when ready, top with the tasty toms.

As an alternative, you can omit the cottage cheese and instead use ½ an avocado and a sprinkling of pine nuts.

Melon, Cheese and Crispbread

This makes a quick and portable breakfast. Grab a cappuccino on the way to work and you're there!

Serves 1

50g feta cheese (in oil rather than vacuum
    packed, as it has a lower sodium
    content)
1 thick slice cantaloupe melon or half a
    small melon
2 crispbreads

Info per serving:
Calories: 176
Carbohydrate: 13g
Protein: 9g
Fat: 10g

Drain the cheese on kitchen paper. Enjoy the ripe melon followed by the crispbreads and cheese.

Berry Berry Crunchy Yoghurt
Serves 1

Handful each of strawberries, raspberries
    and blueberries (about 150g in total)
125g organic natural bio yoghurt
1 tablespoon wheatgerm
2 tablespoons high-fibre muesli

Info per serving:
Calories: 177
Carbohydrate: 28g
Protein: 9g
Fat: 3g

Cut the strawberries in half and place in a bowl with the
other fruit. Stir in the yoghurt and wheat germ. Sprinkle
on the crunchy muesli.

Boiled Egg and Toast with a Virgin Bloody Mary

There is something very nice about enjoying a Bloody
Mary with a leisurely Sunday brunch, but if you ditch
the vodka you can enjoy this favourite every day of the
week and give yourself a health boost at the same time.
Tomatoes are rich in beta-carotene and lycopene, a powerful antioxidant that has been shown to have a protective
effect against prostate cancer.

Serves 1

1 large egg
1 slice thin wholemeal bread
330ml can tomato juice

Info per serving:
Calories: 173
Carbohydrate: 32g
Protein: 7g
Fat: 3g

Tabasco
½ fresh lemon
Black pepper
I celery stick

Boil the egg and toast the bread to your liking. Pour the tomato juice into a tall glass, add a squeeze of lemon juice, a drop of Tabasco, and black pepper to taste and stir with the celery stick. Enjoy your toast and boiled egg as you sip your Virgin Mary and crunch your celery.

SUMMER LUNCHES

Houmous and Salad Pitta Pocket
Serves 4

For the houmous
400g can chickpeas, drained
I tablespoon tahini
Juice of I lemon
125g natural yoghurt (Greek 0% fat
    yogurt by Total is great)
Crushed garlic (lots!)
I tablespoon olive oil
Salt and pepper

A pinch of turmeric
I tablespoon chopped fresh parsley

Info per serving:
Calories: 65
Carbohydrate: 10g
Protein: 3g
Fat: 2g

1 small wholemeal pitta bread
A handful of rocket or watercress
1 small carrot, grated
½ small red chilli, chopped or to taste
A few cherry tomatoes, chopped
6 pitted black olives

Blend all the ingredients for the houmous in a blender until fairly smooth. Sprinkle with the turmeric and chopped parsley. (The houmous will keep in the fridge for a few days.)

Warm the pitta bread, slice open and spread both sides with the houmous. Fill with the rocket or watercress, carrot, chopped fresh chilli, chopped cherry tomatoes and black olives.

Choose your lettuce wisely

Swap iceberg lettuce for darker-leaved varieties, such as cos (often now called romaine). All lettuce leaves are rich in folate, recently shown to be an important cancer-fighting vitamin, but cos is far higher in potassium, contains twice as much fibre as iceberg and is rich in beta-carotene, which pale-leaved lettuces don't contain.

Open Nutty Chicken and Watercress Sandwich

I love this combo, the peanut butter makes it taste rich and naughty but it's incredibly good for you.

Serves I

1 slice thin wholemeal bread
½ tablespoon peanut butter
Handful of watercress
1 cooked chicken breast or leftover roast
    chicken (no skin)
½ teaspoon olive oil
¼ fresh lemon

> **Info per serving:**
> Calories: 238
> Carbohydrate: 16g
> Protein: 21g
> Fat: 11g

Spread the bread with the peanut butter, place the watercress on top and finish with the chopped chicken breast. Drizzle with the olive oil and squeeze over some lemon juice.

Speedy Chilled Pea Soup with Savoury Cottage Cheese

Serves 2

1 small onion, finely chopped
1 teaspoon olive oil
200g bag frozen peas
425ml vegetable stock
Fresh coriander to taste (or coriander
    paste from a tube to save time)

> **Info per serving:**
> Calories: 186
> Carbohydrate: 25g
> Protein: 19g
> Fat: 2g

Salt and pepper
280ml skimmed milk
150g low-fat cottage cheese
2 tomatoes, chopped
Fresh basil leaves
Freshly ground pepper
1 small wholemeal pitta bread

In a large pan, sauté the onion in a little olive oil until soft.
Add the peas, vegetable stock, coriander and seasoning.
Cook for 10 minutes over medium heat. Use a hand
blender to blend the pea stock to your preferred consistency. Add the milk and gently heat through. Allow the
soup to cool then chill it. Meanwhile, mix the cottage
cheese, chopped tomatoes, some basil and black pepper in
a small bowl. Toast the pitta, pour the soup into bowls,
float half a side of the pitta on the soup and add a dollop
of savoury cottage cheese on top. Alternatively, serve the
topped pitta on the side.

Italian Stallion Bean and Tuna Salad
This salad keeps well in the fridge and tastes even better if
left for a day to allow the flavours to develop.

Serves 4

420g can cannellini beans, drained
420g can kidney beans, drained

420g can tuna in spring water, drained
I red onion, finely chopped
Good pinch of Italian herbs
225g can chopped tomatoes
2 tablespoons olive oil
Juice of I fresh lemon or to taste

Info per serving:
Calories: 376
Carbohydrate: 41g
Protein: 43g
Fat: 8g

Mix all the canned ingredients together with the red onion. Add the herbs, tomatoes, olive oil and lemon juice and stir.

This is excellent with toasted pitta bread.

Speedy Gazpacho with Tasty Topping
Serves I

Soup
225g can chopped tomatoes
I small green pepper, seeded
I small red onion, chopped
I teaspoon garlic paste or to taste
Handful fresh basil (or from a tube if fresh
    isn't available)
Good pinch of sugar dissolved in a little hot water
5 ice cubes

Info per serving:
Calories: 353
Carbohydrate: 37g
Protein: 11g
Fat: 20g

Topping
½ avocado, chopped
I hard-boiled egg, chopped

1 tablespoon chopped cucumber
1 small tomato, chopped

Place the canned tomatoes, pepper, red onion, garlic, basil, sugar and ice cubes in a blender. Blend until smooth – you may need to add a little water to stop the blade from sticking. If making in advance, leave this mixture in the fridge to chill. If serving immediately, pour into a wide bowl and top with the avocado, chopped egg, cucumber and tomato.

This is a meal in itself but you may wish to serve it with a small wholemeal roll or top it with squares of wholemeal toast to soak up the lovely juices.

Prawn-stuffed Cucumber Boats
This makes a very attractive lunch, served with a side salad. Alternatively, cut the cucumber in four and eat a quarter as a snack.

Serves 1

100g fresh cooked king prawns
Half cucumber, cut lengthways in half and
    the middle scooped out and reserved
150g natural bio low-fat yoghurt
2 tablespoons cooked brown rice or
    cooked barley
Good handful fresh chopped chives

Info per serving:
Calories: 300
Carbohydrate: 27g
Protein: 21g
Fat: 3g

1 tablespoon lime and coriander sauce (M&S is very good)
Salt and pepper
Flaxseed seasoning (see page 248) to taste

Mix the prawns, cucumber middle, yoghurt, rice, chives, sauce and seasoning to taste in a small bowl. Spoon into the cucumber halves and serve with the flaxseed seasoning sprinkled on top.

CARB CURFEW SUPPERS

Easy Beef Moussaka

This is a simple supper that works well served with a crisp green salad.

Serves 4

3–4 large aubergines, diced
2 small onions, chopped
2 x 400g cans tomatoes (or fresh tomatoes)
500g lean minced beef
50g low-fat grated cheese such as
    Gruyère or reduced-fat Cheddar
Salt and pepper to taste
1–2 tablespoons olive oil

> **Info per serving:**
> Calories: 428
> Carbohydrate: 15g
> Protein: 27g
> Fat: 29g

Heat a tablespoon of olive oil in a large saucepan, add the aubergines and fry, stirring often, until they are thoroughly cooked – you may need to add a little water now and then. Heat the remaining oil in a separate saucepan, add the onions and fry for a few minutes to soften before adding the meat and tomatoes. Cook, stirring and breaking up the meat occasionally, until the meat and onions are cooked – about 25 minutes.

Place a layer of cooked aubergine in the bottom of a large ovenproof dish, top this with a layer of the meat sauce and carry on alternating the ingredients, finishing with a layer of aubergine. Sprinkle the cheese over the top and place under a hot grill for about 5 minutes or until the top is nice and crispy.

Ratatouille Tuna Supper

WORKOUT
WEDGE RECIPE

Ratatouille can be eaten hot or cold, so this can easily be a summer or winter meal.

Serves 2

2 tuna steaks
2–3 large aubergines
1 onion
1 pepper (any colour)
3 medium courgettes
6 tomatoes
1 tablespoon olive oil
1 pinch herbes de Provence
Salt and pepper to taste

Info per serving:
Calories: 325
Carbohydrate: 28g
Protein: 35g
Fat: 10g

Rinse the fish and set aside. Chop all vegetables roughly into cubes. Heat the oil in a large saucepan, add the aubergines and onion and cook over a medium heat for about 10 minutes. Now add the remaining vegetables and herbs along with a small glass of water (not too much as the vegetables will give out a lot of water themselves). Cover and cook on a low heat for about 45 minutes until all the vegetables are soft. Rub a little olive oil into each of the tuna steaks and grill on a hot griddle pan for about 5 minutes, turning once. Cooking time depends on the thickness of the tuna but it should still be a little pink in the middle, so use a very hot griddle. Serve with the rata-touille.

You can make this recipe even simpler by using a can of ready-made ratatouille and adding your own onions or courgettes to make it more substantial.

Cooking vegetables

Vegetables rich in vitamin C and B, such as cruciferous veg-etables and green-leafed veg, benefit from minimal cooking. However, other nutrients, like the cancer-fighting lycopene found in tomatoes and beta-carotene found in carrots, need heat to be released – so don't panic if you overcook these two veg!

Aromatic Summer Salmon with Grape and Chilli Mango Salsa

Serves 2

For the fish:
2 salmon steaks or fillets (or use trout)
1 lemon or lime
Fresh chives or dill

> **Info per serving:**
> Calories: 391
> Carbohydrate: 35g
> Protein: 43g
> Fat: 10g

For the salsa:
1 bunch spring onions, trimmed, sliced small, including some of
    the green parts
1 garlic clove, finely chopped
1 tablespoon grated root ginger
1 mango, cubed fairly small
1 nectarine, cubed (optional)
Small bunch red grapes, cut into halves
1 good handful fresh coriander, chopped
1 good handful fresh mint, chopped
Toasted mixed flax and sesame seeds to taste

Bag of salad (baby spinach and rocket or watercress is particu-
    larly good)
A little red grape juice and lemon juice to dress

You have a choice here – you can either use a steamer or
bake your foil parcels in the oven.

If using a steamer, set the water to boil in the steamer. Rinse the fish under cold running water and pat dry with kitchen paper. Season the fish with a little sea salt, freshly ground black pepper and a good squeeze of lemon or lime juice. Tear off two sheets of foil big enough to contain the fillets. Lightly oil the foil and make a little bed of chives or dill and top each with a salmon steak or fillet. Top with more herbs if wished, and squeeze over a little more lemon or lime juice. Loosely crimp the edges of the foil to seal and place both parcels in the steamer tray. Steam for approximately 15 minutes until the flesh is firm and opaque.

To cook the parcels in the oven, set the oven to 200°C/400°F/Gas mark 6 and bake for 15 minutes.

While the salmon is cooking, mix all the ingredients for the salsa, adding more herbs and some salt and pepper if necessary, and set aside to allow the flavours to develop.

To serve, cover each of the serving plates with the salad leaves. Heap a good serving of salsa in the middle and top with the hot steamed salmon (or it could be served cold if you wish). Finally, sprinkle with some grape juice and lemon.

Tip

To save time, buy ready-poached salmon. The salmon also works well cold so you could prepare this ahead of time, do a workout wedge and then eat your dinner.

Chicken and Aubergine Supper

This is a really simple summer barbecue supper – it looks great and everyone loves the aubergine.

Serves 2

2 chicken breasts

Flaxseed seasoning (see page 248)

2 tablespoons olive oil

125ml white wine

1 aubergine, thinly sliced lengthways

1 garlic clove, sliced in two

Bag of salad leaves

1 tablespoon balsamic vinegar

> **Info per serving:**
> Calories: 286
> Carbohydrate: 10g
> Protein: 29g
> Fat: 10g

Place the chicken breasts in a bowl, sprinkle with a little flaxseed seasoning, drizzle with some olive oil and pour the wine over. Cover and leave to one side. Meanwhile, brush a little olive oil on each slice of aubergine and rub the cut sides of garlic clove into the aubergine flesh.

Heat a barbecue or grill and cook the aubergine slices until they go crispy, turning to brown them on both sides. Place the slices on a piece of kitchen roll to drain and leave to one side.

Now cook the chicken breasts, turning them as they brown and basting them in the marinade. When cooked, remove from the heat.

Mix the balsamic vinegar with a little olive oil and

coat a salad bowl with the mixture. Add the salad leaves and toss. (This method gives the leaves a more even coating.) Serve the salad with the chicken and aubergine slices.

Homemade Burgers with Tomato and Cucumber Salad

Serves 4

450g lean minced beef
1 teaspoon garlic purée
1 teaspoon coriander purée
2 eggs (use only yolk of one)
2 tablespoons cooked plain couscous
Salt and pepper
Flour
400g cherry tomatoes
1 large cucumber
400g can chopped tomatoes
Pinch of sugar dissolved in warm water
Pinch of mixed Italian herbs
Bag of salad leaves
A little olive oil and lemon juice to dress the leaves

> **Info per serving:**
> Calories: 365
> Carbohydrate: 22g
> Protein: 25g
> Fat: 20g

In a large bowl, mix together the minced beef, garlic purée, coriander purée, 2 egg whites and 1 egg yolk, couscous and seasoning. Sprinkle a little flour on a plate.

Take small amounts of the beef mixture and roll in the flour to help shape them. Flatten them into burger shapes, place on a tray and set aside in the fridge to help them hold their shape.

Next chop the cherry tomatoes and cucumber so they are a similar size. Place in a bowl along with the canned tomatoes and mix all three together. Add the dissolved sugar and the herbs and set aside. Light the barbecue or grill and cook the burgers until done on each side. Coat a salad bowl with some lemon juice and olive oil, add the salad and toss. (This method gives the leaves a more even coating.) Serve with the burgers and tomato and cucumber salad.

Tip

If you normally like your burger in a bap, sandwich it between two large cos lettuce leaves instead and add your choice of toppings.

Prawn and Watermelon Salad

This looks really impressive but is quick and simple to assemble. You can find really cheap watermelons at fruit and vegetable markets and buying frozen prawns saves pennies too.

Serves 4

¼ large watermelon
1 lemon

1½ tablespoons extra virgin olive oil

2 tablespoons minced shallot

Salt and pepper

16 king prawns (about 400g), peeled and butterflied (or buy ready-prepared ones for speed)

2 teaspoons ground coriander

125g watercress

125g red leaf lettuce

1 avocado, peeled and cut into 8 slices

Info per serving:
Calories: 205
Carbohydrate: 9g
Protein: 18g
Fat: 12g

Remove the rind from the watermelon, cut the watermelon into chunky cubes and put the fruit in a colander set over a large bowl. Leave for 5 minutes to collect the juice. Remove enough zest from the lemon to make 2 teaspoons and squeeze the juice from it. In a large bowl, blend 2 tablespoons of the lemon juice with olive oil, shallot and lemon zest. Add 2 tablespoons of the watermelon juice and season to taste. Add more watermelon juice if the dressing is too tart. Set aside.

Sprinkle the prawns with the coriander and season on both sides with salt and pepper. Spray a large non-stick sauté pan with cooking spray. Add prawns and sauté over medium-high heat until just cooked, about 2–3 minutes. (If using pre-cooked prawns cut the cooking time.)

Meanwhile, mix the watercress and lettuce and toss with the dressing. Add the watermelon and avocado and toss gently. Divide among four plates and top with the prawns. Serve while the prawns are still warm.

Middle Eastern Chicken

My friend Noelle inspired me to create this dish – she loves Moroccan cooking, so I used some of her favourite ingredients. It's dead simple and is ready in just 10 minutes.

Serves 2

2 cooked boneless chicken breasts (about 130g each), without skin

115g can chickpeas, drained and rinsed

4 medium tomatoes, chopped

2 celery sticks, chopped

I large handful parsley, chopped

2 large handfuls coriander (reserve a little to sprinkle over at the end), chopped

Bag of salad leaves

I orange, peeled and segmented

> **Info per serving:**
> Calories: 458
> Carbohydrate: 31g
> Protein: 52g
> Fat: 17g

Dressing

125g low-fat natural yoghurt

I dessertspoon tahini

½ teaspoon chilli oil (use olive oil if you don't like the heat)

Juice of I orange

Black pepper to taste

½ teaspoon ground mixed spices

½ teaspoon garlic purée

Chop the chicken breasts into cubes, place in a bowl and add the chickpeas, tomatoes, celery, parsley and coriander.

Now mix all the dressing ingredients together until smooth. You can use a hand whisk but I always find the blender easier. Pour the dressing over the prepared chicken mixture and stir so all the ingredients are evenly coated.

Place the salad leaves in a large bowl and arrange the dressed chicken mixture in the centre. Garnish with the orange segments and some chopped coriander.

FIVE-MINUTE CARB CURFEW MEALS

The Carb Curfew meals in the summer and winter plans are mostly quick and pretty easy. However, there are some weeks when you need 'quick' to be virtually immediate! With this in mind, I've put together a collection of five-minute Carb Curfew meals that'll take you through Monday to Friday without taxing your brain, your pocket or your time. The recipes aren't going to impress Gordon Ramsey but they're fast and, what's more, they're rich in fibre and disease-fighting nutrients.

To make life simpler, I have compiled the shopping list for you. The exact quantities you buy will depend how many of you are following the plan so read ahead so you can be fully organized. All you need to do is spend one hour on Monday doing the shopping and you're up and running (though you may want to buy Thursday's and Friday's fresh foods a little later in the week).

The dinners all serve two. Each one comes in at around 400 calories, so you could easily lose weight, especially since many of the dinners we grab on the run when not operating my Carb Curfew can weigh in at more than 700 calories. Oh, and another thing – anyone can cook these recipes, whether you were born with the cooking gene or not!

SHOPPING LIST

Salad greens

Canned salmon

Canned pineapple chunks in natural juice

Canned kidney beans (preferably in unsalted water)

Canned sweetcorn (preferably in unsalted, unsweetened
  water)

Jar of salsa

Cooked roast chicken

Low-fat natural yoghurt

Pre-cut and washed mixed vegetables

Fresh spinach (2 bags)

Fresh tomato or gazpacho soup from chiller cabinet

Onions

Avocado

200g packet frozen mixed seafood – mussels, cockles,
  squid etc.

Eggs

Lean ham

Canned chickpeas

1 can V8 juice

Tuna canned in spring water

Canned white cannellini beans

Cherry tomatoes

Romaine or cos lettuce

Can of minestrone soup

STORE CUPBOARD ESSENTIALS

Olive oil

Balsamic vinegar

Mango chutney

Reduced-calorie French dressing

Cumin

Monday: Salmon Pineapple Platter

Serves 2

Bag of salad greens

213g can salmon

200g can pineapple chunks in own juice

2 teaspoons olive oil

4 teaspoons balsamic vinegar

180g can red kidney beans, drained

165g can sweetcorn, drained

Info per serving:
Calories: 370
Carbohydrate: 51g
Protein: 37g
Fat: 15g

100g salsa
Pinch of cumin

1. Divide the salad greens between the two plates.
2. Place half the salmon on the side of each plate.
3. Place half the pineapple on the other side of the plate.
4. Mix the olive oil and vinegar together and drizzle over the two plates.
5. Combine the kidney beans, sweetcorn and salsa with the cumin and spoon into the middle of the salad.

Tuesday: Instant Roasted Coronation Chicken

Serves 2

90g bag pre-cut mixed vegetables
2 tablespoons mango chutney
125g low-fat natural yoghurt
250g cooked chicken breast from deli
     counter or supermarket chill cabinet
100g microwave-in-the-bag spinach

> **Info per serving:**
> Calories: 286
> Carbohydrate: 11g
> Protein: 45g
> Fat: 5g

1. Place the vegetables in a microwave to cook or cook in boiling water.
2. Mix the mango chutney and yoghurt and leave to one side.
3. If you like your chicken warm, heat it a little in the microwave.

4. Divide the spinach between two plates and place the chicken on top. Spoon the coronation yoghurt sauce over the top.
5. Serve with the mixed veg.

Wednesday: Fancy Mediterranean Soup Supper

Serves 2

1 small onion, finely chopped
1 teaspoon olive oil
600ml carton fresh tomato or gazpacho
    soup from chill cabinet
200g packet frozen mixed seafood
    (mussels, cockles, squid), defrosted
½ an avocado

> **Info per serving:**
> Calories: 255
> Carbohydrate: 15g
> Protein: 16g
> Fat: 15g

1. Sauté the onion in the olive oil until nearly soft.
2. Add the soup and mixed seafood and heat thoroughly.
3. Slice the avocado while the soup is being heated.
4. Divide the soup between two bowls and top with the sliced avocado.

Sweet tooth? Have one small scoop of ice cream.

Thursday: Wilted Spinach and Ham Omelette

Serves 2

100g bag ready-to-cook spinach

5 eggs

3 tablespoons skimmed milk

Salt and pepper

½ tablespoon olive oil

125g can chickpeas

50g lean ham

1 tablespoon grated reduced-fat Cheddar cheese

330ml can V8 juice

Info per serving:
Calories: 344
Carbohydrate: 21g
Protein: 27g
Fat: 17g

1. Place a small cup of boiling water in a large non-stick saucepan. Add the spinach, cover and cook for 2 minutes or until the spinach starts to wilt. Remove the lid and turn up the heat so the remaining water evaporates. Drain and squeeze out any remaining water if necessary.
2. Beat the eggs, then add the milk and seasoning.
3. Heat the oil in a non-stick omelette pan and add the egg mixture. Tease the spinach apart a little and spread a layer over the eggs. Now sprinkle over the chickpeas.
4. Heat through until the egg starts to set on the bottom, then sprinkle on the ham and cheese. Flip one half of the omelette over the other just before the egg is set – this helps the cheese to melt.
5. Serve with the V8 juice.

Friday: Tuna Lettuce Parcels

Serves 2

400g can minestrone soup

212g can tuna in spring water, drained

420g can cannellini beans, drained

113g can sweetcorn and peppers in water,
    drained

3 tablespoons reduced-calorie French
    dressing

1 tablespoon low-fat natural yoghurt

100g cos or romaine lettuce

6 cherry tomatoes, quartered

Info per serving:
Calories: 399
Carbohydrate: 47g
Protein: 36g
Fat: 6g

1. Heat the soup gently.
2. Mix together the tuna, cannellini beans and sweetcorn.
3. Mix together the French dressing and natural yoghurt and
   add to the bean and tuna mixture.
4. Arrange the lettuce leaves on the plates.
5. Spoon the bean mixture into the middle of the lettuce
   and sprinkle with the tomatoes.
6. Eat the soup and enjoy the tuna and bean mix, using the
   lettuce as scoops.

Sweet tooth? Finish with an apple and a tablespoon of
peanut butter.

DROP A SIZE FOR LIFE FOODS

More and more evidence is coming to light about how certain nutrients in specific foods can positively improve our health – and in particular reduce the risk of cardiovascular disease. These foods are often referred to as 'functional' foods. As you are already aware, dropping a size for life will reduce your risk of certain diseases, but incorporating certain functional foods into your diet will also improve your health and reduce your health risks in other areas, too.

Some functional foods are not what you might think appropriate for a 'diet', however, you can enjoy them on the Drop a Size for Life plan. In fact, you might like to think of this plan as your 'heart-protective' diet, too. Research has shown that individuals can reduce their risk of cardiovascular disease by eating specific amounts of the following types of functional foods: tea, oats, nuts, grapes, flaxseed, fatty fish, psyllium, soy, and cholesterol-lowering margarines. The specific amount of each food needed to boost heart health is referred to as 'the effective daily intake'. Each of the foods is discussed below, with tips on how to incorporate them into your Drop a Size for Life plan, and on pages 250–51 you'll find a table for quick reference.

What are Functional Foods?

The American Dietetic Association defines functional foods as having '… a potentially beneficial effect on health when consumed as part of a varied diet, on a regular basis, at effective levels' – this can include whole, fortified, enriched or enhanced foods.

Functional foods are intended to enhance your Drop a Size for Life eating habits. However, total calories are still important so don't fall into the trap of thinking that just because these foods are good for you, you get a greater benefit by eating more of them!

⌒⌒ OATS

Oats lower cholesterol thanks to the soluble fibre beta-glucan. In addition, research shows that they may even improve the ratio of good (HDL) to bad (LDL) cholesterol.

What's the best source?: Instant oatmeal, rolled oats, oat bran and whole oat flour are all good sources. See page 198 for a protein-powered porridge recipe.

How much should I have?: The effective daily intake is 3g of oat soluble fibre. This is equivalent to approximately 1 cup of cooked oat bran, 1½ cups of cooked porridge or 3 cups of oat-based cereal such as Cheerios.

Tip

Oats also boost your energy for longer. As a low to moderate glycaemic-loaded carbohydrate, porridge oats or oat-based cereals make a great breakfast as they give a slow release of energy, helping to curb mid-morning snack attacks!

⌒⌒ TEA

Yes, the good old British cuppa is good for you. Tea contains natural antioxidants that may play an important role in maintaining optimal health. Tea decreases the stickiness of blood, reducing the risk of blood clots. Consuming one to two cups of green or black tea daily may be a prudent way to boost heart health.

What's the best way to enjoy it?: Simple – put the kettle on, put your feet up and let it brew! If you haven't already done so, you may want to try green tea for a refreshing change. Your local Chinese restaurant will offer you Jasmine tea after your meal – this is the same as green tea.

How much should I have?: One or two cups of tea per day has been shown to decrease artery clogging by nearly 50 per cent. With four or more cups per day, the reduction was nearly 70 per cent. However, given that black tea can dehydrate the body, those who like more than two cups a day would be better making at least some of these green tea (as this doesn't dehydrate the body).

⚬⚬⚬ NUTS

Nuts are a good source of a number of nutrients that may enhance heart health, including fibre, vitamin E, magnesium and other plant chemicals. In a recent study, researchers found that more frequent nut consumption was associated with a decreased risk of sudden cardiac death and a 30 per cent lower risk of dying from coronary heart disease.

Nuts are also a rich source of the amino acid arginine, which plays a role in maintaining the health and flexibility of arteries.

Where can I get these nutrients?: All nuts, but be adventurous – try various nut butters, such as almond and Brazil butters, as a change from what you usually spread on your toast. Macadamia nuts, pecans and walnuts in particular can lower cholesterol if they are part of a long-term diet.

How much should I have?: Consuming 125g a week has been recognized as the optimum amount.

But I thought nuts were very fattening!

As healthy as nuts are, yes they are high in calories and total fat: 56g of almonds = 332 calories, 56g of walnuts = 344 calories and 56g of pecans = 378 calories, while a tablespoon of peanut butter gives you 95 calories. If you were to add 50g of nuts to your daily diet without compensating for it in any way this could, in theory, mean a gain of 20–35 pounds in weight – equivalent to maybe gaining three dress sizes! So to increase nut consumption you must decrease calories in other areas of your diet. The best way to do this is to substitute nuts and nut butters for equal calories from refined carbohydrates. That way you benefit twice – you get the good stuff, plus you miss out on refined carbs, such as white bread, which can increase your risk of diabetes.

Easy switches

- Substitute 1 tablespoon sliced almonds for 1 tablespoon of low-fibre cereal such as cornflakes.
- Ditch 1 tablespoon of your cooked lunchtime pasta in favour of 1 tablespoon of pistachios.
- Instead of having a handful of croutons on your salad, try 1 tablespoon of chopped walnuts.

⌐⊃ SOY PROTEIN

Soy has a number of health properties. It helps blood vessels stay flexible, which lowers the risk of blockages from clots, and it has been found to significantly lower both total and LDL cholesterol (that's the bad one associated with increased risk of heart attacks).

Where can I find it?: Soy protein is found naturally in soy milk, tofu, tempeh, roasted soy nuts and miso.

How much should I have?: The effective daily intake of soy protein is 25g a day.

Tip

Add soy protein to your diet gradually; if it is added too quickly some people experience indigestion, wind and bloating. This is most likely because of the dietary fibre in soy. Start out with one serving of soy food a day and work up to two to three servings to reach the effective daily intake of 25g.

Make your own soy 'mayo'

Use natural tofu or low soya fat yoghurt as the base and add wholegrain mustard, tomato ketchup, mango chutney – or whatever flavouring you enjoy.

⌐⊃ RED GRAPES

Good news – researchers have linked wine intake to a reduced risk of cardiovascular disease in both men and women. The health benefits of wine have been attributed in part to the high concentration of antioxidants in grapes, which are thought to help relax blood vessels and reduce the thickness of the blood.

If you don't like alcohol, you can reap the benefits from fresh grapes instead. Research carried out at Glasgow University found that red grapes offer higher levels of antioxidants than white grapes. Red grapes are packed with polyphenols (antioxidants that are believed to help reduce heart disease risk) and ellagic acid, a phytochemical that may have cancer-fighting properties. All grapes – white and red – are a good source of vitamin C and fibre.

Where can I get the benefits?: From red wine, grape juice or grapes.

How much is beneficial?: One glass a day for women and two for men (see God really is a man!), or two cups of grapes.

Does all fruit juice have the same effect?

No! In a study that compared grape, orange and grapefruit juice consumption, only grape juice was found to reduce the stickiness of blood, a factor that contributes to heart attack. So for a change, why not swap your morning glass of OJ for a glass of grape juice or switch your orange for a small bunch of grapes?

⌒⌒ PSYLLIUM

Psyllium is another soluble fibre shown to be very effective in lowering blood cholesterol levels. This fibre is especially rich in the husk of the psyllium seed.

Where do I get it?: Psyllium seed husk can be obtained in bulk form in natural food stores. Once it is ground, add the powder to juices, smoothies or cooked cereals.

How much should I have?: The effective daily intake required to significantly reduce serum lipids is 7g. This amount would be expected to reduce total cholesterol by 4–6 per cent and decrease LDL cholesterol by 4–8 per cent.

Tip

It's best to consume your psyllium with liquid as blockages in the gut can occur if psyllium seed husk is consumed with insufficient liquid.

⌒⌒ FATTY FISH

Fatty fish and their oils are good sources of the omega-3 fatty acids. The oils appear to reduce blood triglycerides and hence have great heart-protective effects. This explains why Greenland Eskimos, whose diet is rich in fish, have exceptionally low rates of heart disease. Scientists also believe that the severe lack of omega-3 fatty acids in our modern diet helps explain the rising rates of depression in the 21st century.

What kind of fish should I look for?: Fatty fish or cold water fish such as mackerel, herring, sardines, salmon and tuna.
How much should I eat?: At least two servings of fatty fish each week (75–150g per serving).

Tip

Prepare your fish without adding saturated fat, as this will only undo the potential benefit. If you must add oil then use olive or canola oil, which are high in monounsaturated fats.

Canned Tuna

When buying canned tuna choose water-packed white tuna as opposed to the light meat tuna. Water-packed tuna has the most omega-3 fats.

STEROL- AND STANOL-ENRICHED MARGARINE

Certain plant-derived components called plant sterols and stanols resemble cholesterol, which allows them to compete with bad cholesterol during digestion inside the body. Recent studies have shown that plant sterols and stanols decrease blood cholesterol levels.
Where can I get it?: Benecol and Flora Proactive are two types of this margarine that are widely available in supermarkets. Other hard block brands, suitable for baking, are more widely available in health food stores.

How much should I have?: 2–3 grams a day of these substances has been shown to decrease LDL cholesterol by 9–20 per cent. This equates to about 2 tablespoons of sterol- or stanol-enriched margarine.

Típ

Team cholesterol-cutting spreads with orange or green vegetables and fruits. These are rich in beta-carotene, a vital nutrient that is depleted, along with the bad cholesterol, by the cholesterol-lowering margarines. Try sweet potato, broccoli, carrots and cantaloupe melon.

Flavoured margarines

A very good standby, when you're in a hurry and want to jazz up some plain vegetables, grilled white fish, chicken breast or a pork chop, is a ready-to-use flavoured 'log' made with these enriched margarines. Simply cream or beat in additions such as garlic, herbs, spices, grated lemon zest, or minced spring onion and add to your chosen food.

FLAXSEED

Flaxseed contains significant amounts of the essential fatty acid omega-3, as well as lignans, a type of phytoestrogen. Eating the entire seed appears to have the greatest overall health benefit. Flaxseed is high in fibre and, since it has a laxative effect, should be added to the diet gradually. Flaxseed also has benefits for cancer prevention.

Where can I find it?: Flaxseed is widely available in health food stores.

How do I use it?: Ground flaxseed meal may be used in baking (muffins, breads, etc.) sprinkled on cereal, added to fruit drinks or smoothies, or even mixed with peanut butter or soy nut butter and used as a spread.

How much should I have?: Start with 1 to 2 teaspoons of ground flax meal per day and work up to 2 tablespoons (1 tablespoon of ground flax equals approximately 8g).

Tip

You can buy whole seeds and grind them yourself in a coffee grinder. Grinding them helps release the essential fats, thus aiding your body to obtain the nutrients. Grind a batch in one go and then store in a tightly-sealed container in the fridge.

Flaxseed seasoning

One exciting way of incorporating flaxseed into your meals is to create your own tailor-made spiced seasoning for cooking. The following recipe will give a burst of exciting flavours to your cooking and reduce or replace the need for salt. This mixture works particularly well rubbed into chicken for the barbecue, or try it with chops or fish (with a dash of lemon) when pan frying or grilling. Quick and easy to prepare, this quantity will keep you going for a few weeks – and stored in an airtight container, will keep its flavour well.

What you need
1 tablespoon coriander seeds
1 tablespoon cumin seeds
1 tablespoon fennel seeds
about 4 tablespoons ground flaxseed
about 4 tablespoons crushed dried sea vegetable

What you do
Dry fry the coriander, cumin and fennel seeds in a hot pan over a medium heat. Keep gently shaking the pan until the seeds release their spicy aroma – take care not to scorch or burn the seeds. Grind the cooled seeds and combine with an equal quantity of ground flaxseed and add crushed dried sea vegetable to taste.

Variations
Experiment with your favourite spices to create more or less flavour and piquancy – for example, add celery salt, smoked paprika, chilli flakes, ginger, etc. You can also combine equal quantities of dried herbs and ground flaxseed to use as a flavouring for omelettes or roasting vegetables.

DROP A SIZE FOR LIFE FOODS

Food	The bit that makes it extra healthy	Effective daily intake	Examples
soy	soy protein	25g	½ cup tofu = 10g ½ cup cooked soybeans = 11g ¼ cup roasted soy nuts = 15g 1 cup fortified soy milk = 10g ¼ cup soy protein, dry =11g
oats	beta-glucan	3g	1 cup cooked oat bran 1½ cups cooked oatmeal 3 cups Cheerios
psyllium	psyllium fibre	7g	10g psyllium, ground seed & husk
flaxseed	essential fatty acids & fibre	15–50g	1 tbsp ground flaxseed = 8g

Food	The bit that makes it extra healthy	Effective daily intake	Examples
tea	antioxidants	1–2 cups	brewed tea (green or black)
nuts	mono-unsaturated fatty acids	30–55g	approx. 3 tbsp = 30g nuts
red grapes	antioxidants	1–2 cups juice 140ml red wine (women) 280ml red wine (men)	red grapes red grape juice red wine
fatty fish	omega-3 fatty acids	at least 2 servings per week	1 serving = 85–160g (tuna, salmon, herring, mackerel, sardines)
cholesterol-lowering margarines	plant-based sterols & stanols	1.3g sterols (e.g. Take Control) 3.4g stanols (e.g. Benecol)	2 tbsp

TROUBLESHOOTING:
SOME COMMONLY ASKED
QUESTIONS AND PROBLEMS

'I still feel hungry when I've finished eating'

Are you sure? Go back to step 1 in section one to remind yourself of the action points for improving mind-body awareness. Many of us simply eat without paying any attention to what we're doing and then feel we haven't actually had the experience and hence don't feel satiated.

In a Swedish study, subjects who were blindfolded ate 22 per cent less calories than usual but reported feeling just as full. The theory behind this is that many of us rely on visual external cues as a prompt for hunger or satisfaction. For example, an empty plate has associations with a full tummy but a plate that has some food left on it may convince us that we are still hungry!

Short of blindfolding yourself, here are some practical ways to tune into your body's hunger clues and eat less:

- Clear the table
  Place the mail and other clutter elsewhere and set the table
  with the dinnerware and a candle or table decoration.
- Avoid distractions
  Don't watch TV or read a magazine while eating.
  Distractions mean you are less likely to notice when you
  are comfortably full.
- Go solo
  Eating alone allows you to notice when you're full. If that's
  not practical, limit your number of dinner companions.
- Serve individual courses
  Serve your salad first then have your main course. This will
  make your meal experience longer, giving you more time
  to register you are full.
- Close your eyes
  Even for a few bites, closing your eyes will help you focus
  on the food and tastes you are experiencing.

'I have started exercising and have gained a size'

It is fantastic you have started exercising, so don't be put
off by this – it's probably just down to one of a number
of teething problems that are common with people who
are new to exercise. Address these issues and you'll soon
find yourself back on track:

- **Too much refuelling**

  Many exercisers misguidedly scoff their way through energy bars, health bars or drinks, under the misconception that they have burnt off enough calories to justify this. A good proportion of recovery bars and energy drinks are more appropriate for elite athletes who regularly expend 600–1000 calories per training day. The average individual at the gym will be more likely to expend 300–400 calories max. In addition, many people think they contain a magical ingredient to improve strength and muscle growth whereas in reality they are packed with calories. So beware of these products – they can load on the calories and result in you gaining a size rather than losing one.

  If you really do feel you need to refuel after a workout, opt for a simple piece of fruit or a handful of dried fruit and nuts and a glass of water. Try to keep it to 150 calories, which will still leave you with a calorie deficit.

Case Study: Richard's Story

Richard, the MD of a record label and a client of mine, was really making progress with his running training. He also swore blind he was operating the Carb Curfew, and his wife confirmed this, but he was still not losing pounds. One day, after a training session, Richard offered me a drink and when he returned with my glass of water he was also carrying a high-energy drink weighing in at 450 calories – I now knew where he was going wrong!

- **A 'once and done' attitude**

  Many people think that doing 30 minutes on the treadmill
  gives them the opportunity to take the lift, the escalator
  and park the car nearest to the shops. However, exercise
  is cumulative. The more physically active you are, even
  when you are not 'exercising', the better the result you'll
  experience (see in section two pages 115–118 for more
  information on how you can exercise without even
  putting on your trainers). Your body is meant to move a
  lot so avoid thinking of exercise as something you do for
  30 minutes a day only.

- **Driven to distraction**

  Watching TV or listening to your favourite track as you
  exercise can be a good thing to keep you on a piece of
  equipment, but if you're so engrossed in reading the latest
  celeb gossip mag that your legs are only going around at a
  half pace on the bicycle, you're only kidding yourself. Use
  that mag for your warm up and cool down as a reward to
  get you there into the gym in the first place. In the main
  body of your workout, try to engage in your workout and
  focus on performing the exercise well and your intensity –
  high energy exercise can be great in this respect, as it
  requires you to stay focussed.

- **Don't treat yourself with food**

  Building in a reward system for your exercise efforts is
  vital, but that reward doesn't need to be food. Using food
  in this way often results in you eating more calories than
  you have expended. If you're going to use a great dinner

or gooey dessert as a reward for your physical efforts then reward yourself less frequently – once a fortnight, not every day. For more frequent rewards opt for make-up, CDs, a beauty treatment or massage, clothes or other non-food items.

'I practically live on salad, but I'm not losing weight.'

Even if most of your meals are salads, are they made up predominantly of salad leaves and other water-packed vegetables like cucumber, celery and tomatoes, or are they bulked up with pasta or rice and swimming in mayonnaise or calorie-laden dressing? We often think of salads as packed with vegetables but many of the pre-prepared salads in shops are laden with carbohydrate without a single serving of vegetables. In addition, some of the layered salads that are particularly popular in summer as one-pot lunches can total up to a whopping 600–950 calories in one hit. One example – a shop-bought, layered cheese salad – packs in 980 calories and 72g of fat and is sold as a single serving! Salad doesn't need to be boring to be healthy – you can add nuts and seeds, roasted veg (mushrooms and peppers work particularly well) and experiment with your own homemade dressings. So the message is read the labels.

A FEW TIPS

- If you normally make a traditional French dressing, use half the amount of oil and vinegar and fill with water (for a runnier dressing) or natural yoghurt for a creamy, lower-fat alternative. **This is my recipe for a healthy salad dressing:**

  50ml balsamic or white wine vinegar
  2 teaspoons olive oil
  2 teaspoons Dijon mustard
  1 garlic clove, crushed
  Juice of half a lemon
  1 teaspoon runny honey
  1 tablespoon natural yoghurt (optional)

  Combine all the ingredients in a screw-top jar and shake vigorously to combine. Add water to make the dressing go further.

- When you serve a salad, use a sharp knife to cut through the leaves and other ingredients to release their moisture. This will enable you to go easy on the dressing.
- Coat your salad bowl with a little of the dressing first before adding the salad leaves and then toss. You get a more even dressing on your salad, plus it will go further saving you extra calories.
- Watch out for salad bars. Whether you've got a salad shop just round the corner from your office or you're

tempted by the supermarket salad bar, practice a bit of restraint. Yes they're so convenient and a really accessible way to get your daily five portions of fruits and vegetables, but it's very tempting to eat oversized portions and pack your box with high-fat, calorie-dense salads. Eating healthy doesn't mean you can eat more! The best advice I can give is load up the carton first with all the water-packed vegetables, add a serving of proteins – nuts, tuna or ham and then top with a little of the rice or pasta and more fattening dressed salads.

'I hate fruit and vegetables – can't I get my nutrients from vitamin pills instead?'

No. Vitamin pills are not a replacement for a healthy, nutritious diet with lots of fruit and vegetables. There are all kinds of micronutrients in fruit and veg – such as cancer-fighting phytochemicals – that cannot be manufactured. Scientists also believe that they have so far discovered only a fraction of the micronutrients that influence our health. However, due to growing stress levels, eating on the go and the high consumption of processed foods, a multivitamin can be a safeguard for us all – but it certainly shouldn't be a replacement for a balanced diet.

The answer is to learn to love your fruit and veg. Here are some tips to help you on your way.

• Don't overcook vegetables. Soft, mushy carrots and broccoli are reminiscent of school dinners and enough to put anyone off! Ideally, use a steamer and only cook the vegetables until they are 'al dente'.

- Experiment with stir-frying vegetables in a little soy sauce to add flavour. It doesn't have to be beansprouts and baby corn, 'traditional' English vegetables like carrots, courgettes and leeks taste just as good.

- Go exotic! For many of us, fruit means apples, oranges and bananas. What about mangoes, pineapple, kiwi fruit, rhubarb, strawberries, nectarines, papaya, apricots, watermelon, cantaloupe, figs and wonderful antioxidant-rich blueberries, blackberries and redcurrants? Make the most of what is in season and you'll get it at its best.

- Try some new and unusual vegetables, too. Make a pledge to put something new from the vegetable aisle in your supermarket trolley every week. Try celeriac, fennel, pak choi, aubergine. Or experiment with cooking your usual veg in a different way.

- If the idea of all that chopping and peeling puts you off, invest in your health by opting for ready-prepared fruit, salad and veg, or ensure you have more of them when you're eating out, when someone else is doing the preparing!

'I've tried to get the kids involved but they just aren't interested. Should I force them to exercise?'
It isn't a good idea to force your children to do activities they aren't keen on. You might think a family bike ride is great, but they might not, so try to find other activities

that they will enjoy – offer them a choice. A recent study showed that being forced to exercise during the preteen years had a negative impact on individuals taking up exercise as an adult.

The trick is to persevere – don't give into the GameBoy just yet! Many parents may imagine that watching TV or playing video games has minimal impact as long as these activities are time limited. However, the evidence indicates that these sedentary pastimes not only have a negative physical impact, they can also affect your child's mood. Studies have shown that the same amount of time spent in physical activity boosts children's moods and decreases their negative feelings compared to watching TV. Why not try the Playground Workout Wedge on page 130?

'Surely if I exercise enough, I don't have to diet?'

It's true that the more exercise you do, the more calories you'll expend on a daily basis. However, study after study has shown that for successful weight loss and maintenance of that weight loss, exercise and a healthy diet must both be addressed. You may have a certain amount of success with exercise alone but your efforts will be far more richly rewarded if you combine exercise with good dietary habits.

As we learned in Fundamental four, structured workouts are a great way of improving aerobic fitness, strength and flexibility, but they aren't the be-all and end-all of physical activity. Even a high intensity hour (such as running or a kickboxercise class) can only burn an average of 400–500 calories, so unless you are doing that amount daily, along with being generally active, it isn't going to be sufficient to help you drop that size.

One final thought: even if you are immensely active, it doesn't mean you can eat whatever you like and still be healthy. The usual rules of healthy nutrition still apply.

'My job entails eating out a lot. How can I avoid weight gain?'

When eating out is an integral part of your lifestyle, you need to develop some strategies to help you avoid regular calorie overload. Nutritionists reckon that the average person eating out at a restaurant consumes a whole day's calorie intake in one sitting, so it's easy to see how that translates into an expanding waistline.

Here are some tips to help you eat out without gaining a size:

- As far as possible always operate the Carb Curfew.
- Stick to one course – or have a very light starter and main course.
- Avoid the breadbasket (and especially the butter!)
- Fill up on salads – ask for the dressing to be brought on the side so you can use just a little.
- Avoid cream- and cheese-based sauces on your food.
- Opt for baked, grilled or roasted dishes rather than fried ones.
- Choose fish, poultry or lean cuts of meat.

- Avoid pies and pastry-based dishes.
- Ask for vegetables, even if they aren't specified on the menu.
- Go easy on the alcohol. Ask for a bottle of water to be brought to the table so you don't guzzle wine thoughtlessly.
- Select from the menu before you drink your wine – you'll make a more sensible choice at this stage.
- Go to the restaurant with a couple of ideas of what healthy foods you would like to eat – this will help guide your choices and stop you being tempted by other things.

For those of us for whom eating out is a special treat, there's no need to worry about every single thing we put in our mouths. Remember, the 80-20 rule states that as long as we do the right thing 80 per cent of the time, the remaining 20 per cent of the time is when we can enjoy life to the full. Look back at pages 182–188 for more advice on this.

'Are there any supplements I can take to help me lose weight?'

Wouldn't it be great if all our weight loss needs could be met by a magic pill? Well, science's best efforts haven't yet produced that pill, although that doesn't prevent a multi-million pound industry selling diet pills, slimming aids and supplements by the billion. A lot of the natural supplements available will only play a very minor part in helping you to drop a size. It must be stressed that they are no substitute for applying the 10 fundamentals outlined earlier. The fundamentals will not only help you drop a size and keep that size off but they will also have a huge impact on your health, which medication and supplements alone cannot achieve. In addition, some of the claims made by the manufacturers of diet supplements are not scientifically validated. This means it has not been proven that they are effective on everyone. Yes, they may have worked on some people, but that is not to say they always work on everyone every time. That said, there are some naturally-occurring substances that *may* assist your efforts – if you combine them with the 10 fundamentals.

There is some evidence that green tea increases fat oxidation and daily energy expenditure. One study found that mice fed a diet containing 2 or 4 per cent green tea extract had lower levels of leptin (the appetite-regulating hormone) and less fat accumulation and weight gain than mice that were not fed the green tea. Those who were on a 4 per cent green tea diet also voluntarily ate less food.

Also of interest are lecithin granules, the purest source of soy protein. Lecithin complex is an active nutrient believed to be invaluable in the breakdown of fats. As such, it is a valuable supplement for those following a low cholesterol diet – and clients of mine have found it useful in helping them control their body fat. However, there is little scientific evidence to support its role in weight loss and I include it in this section simply because it has helped a number of my clients.

One supplement to *avoid* is ephedra. Excessive consumption places the user at considerable health risk. Symptoms include increased anxiety, headaches, kidney stones, irregular heartbeat, insomnia, tremors, acute rise in blood pressure, heart attack and stroke. There have even been reports of some deaths associated with it.

'Can my doctor give me any medication to help me drop a size?'
There are several weight loss medications available. However, they are not appropriate to everyone and, where prescribed, they still should be seen as an adjunct to a healthy lifestyle.

Weight-loss drugs work by either preventing the body from absorbing fatty acids in the intestine or inhibiting the break down of fatty acids so they are excreted from the body before they are stored as fat. Xenical (Orlistat) works locally in the gut to reduce dietary fat absorption by around 30 per cent and is the most widely used pharmacological weight loss aid in the world. Research shows that it is not only successful in helping patients lose weight, but also in helping them maintain their weight loss.

In trials, those on Xenical showed:

- More than twice as much weight loss as those on diet alone (6.4kg loss, compared to 2.9kg in those on a placebo).

- A significantly greater reduction in waist measurement compared to those on diet alone (6.1cm vs. 3.8cm).
- Improved blood pressure, triglyceride levels and blood glucose levels.

However – and it's a big however – it has some pretty unpleasant side effects and it's not suitable for everyone. In addition, it is only prescribed to people who are obese (look back at page 7 to work out your BMI), not those who simply want to lose a few pounds.

'I love burger and pizza and all fast food – do I have to give them up to drop a size for life?'

No you don't – if you operate the 80-20 rule you'll still be able to enjoy your favourite fast foods, you'll just have to eat less of them and less frequently. However, in my experience, as people begin to make the fundamentals part of their life, their taste buds change. If you like burgers, how about making your own healthy beef burgers and instead of serving them in a bun, 'bap' them between two large iceburg lettuce leaves. The firmness of the iceburg lettuce supports your burger and if you get a big enough lettuce it can easily hold all your dressing too. Or how about taking your favourite pizza topping and instead of putting it on a pizza base, use a large flat mushroom instead. You save calories, fat and gain an extra serving of vegetables!

KEEPING YOUR NEW SIZE FOR LIFE

INTRODUCTION

Life is a different journey for all of us, but there are certain landmarks along the way that virtually all women pass – for instance, pregnancy and the menopause – and these life changes can impact on weight management and size. Although what triggers these life stages is happening deep inside your body – such as changes in hormone levels, body composition and metabolic rate – there are also many social, environmental and psychological changes that occur at different stages of life. And these can all potentially affect our size and our shape. Having a baby, for example, is very obviously physical, but suddenly having to take care of a new life is likely also to impact on your mental well-being, perhaps leaving you feeling tired and low on self-confidence.

In this section, I'll explain what happens to your body during key life stages. I'll outline the science behind the physiological changes taking place in your body and also examine the other factors likely to be associated with the life stage – the environmental, social, emotional and psychological issues. This will provide you with the navigation tools you need to steer a course through life's individual challenges, with your ideal size intact! You've already achieved so much by dropping a size – now let's stop those rebound pounds!

The way in which you deal with not just these life stages, but your life in general on a daily, weekly, monthly and yearly basis, is crucial to your weight management success. After all, life is just a series of 'now' moments and it's up to you to make the most of them all. That's not to say that you should aim to stick to a precise waist or hip measurement for every day of your life. As we learned in the introduction, successful weight management is about staying within 20 per cent of your goal weight and knowing how to respond to internal or external challenges where necessary.

As we go through each life stage in this section, I'll highlight some of the common hurdles we have to cross if we are to maintain our ideal size. I call this Drop a Size (DAS) management and each life stage has a DAS management plan. Of course, not all the scenarios will apply to you, but you may find them useful in future, or for someone else you know, such as your mother, sister or daughter. You'll also find lots of useful references to sections one and two, so that the action you take is a combination of the mental and physical – which will help you continue to develop a close body–brain relationship. If you are still searching for your G spot motivation, look out for the 'Does this tickle your G spot?' text, which you should find helpful.

LIFE STAGE

THE CHILD-BEARING YEARS

Whether you intend to have a baby or not, during the 30 or so years that is your child-bearing 'window', your body is gearing itself up to have one, which means it is experiencing huge hormonal changes on a monthly basis. These have a bearing on your metabolism, your moods and your energy levels – all of which can have a direct and indirect impact on your eating and exercise patterns and how you feel about yourself.

WHAT'S HAPPING INSIDE YOUR BODY

During the childbearing years, your body will have to deal with some or all of the following: periods, PMS, contraception, conception, pregnancy and giving birth, all of which are accompanied by major hormonal fluctuations. The primary hormones that affect you and your monthly cycle are oestrogen, progesterone and a group of hormones called prostaglandins. The amount of each of these hormones changes at different stages of your cycle, affecting your energy, your metabolism and your moods. Maintaining your ideal size is therefore, in part, about being aware of these hormonal changes, their possible impact and how you can deal with this.

Making sense of the female hormones

The female monthly cycle is a complicated one that is governed by an intricate set of hormones and controlled by a series of clever feedback mechanisms. At the start of your period, levels of oestrogen and progesterone are low then, as a follicle-stimulating hormone is released, causing an egg in the ovaries to ripen, oestrogen is secreted in increasing amounts to enable the womb lining to grow thicker. This is in anticipation of conceiving – the womb is preparing itself to hold a developing baby for nine months. At mid-cycle, normally at around day 14, the egg is released and the amount of oestrogen secreted drops as progesterone levels increase – again in preparation for conception. This premenstrual surge of progesterone boosts metabolic rate and stimulates fluid retention, as your body is preparing itself for change. If conception doesn't take place, the egg degenerates and both hormone levels plummet, leading to a period and a return to normal in metabolic rate and body fluid levels.

YOU ARE . . . YOUNG, FREE AND SINGLE

When life is a social whirl, you're putting in long hours to further your career and you seem to be able to get away with murder in terms of your lifestyle habits, it's easy to assume that you are invincible and that you don't need to worry about developing good eating and exercise habits. Wrong! The action you take now is an investment for keeping your new size for life. However, it doesn't mean ditching your social life – it's merely a case of instilling some good habits now, so that they have become routine by the time you reach your thirties.

Does this tickle your G spot?

Figuring out your future figure

You may have been blessed with a great figure in your twenties but that doesn't necessarily mean you'll keep it. A study in the *Journal of the American Dietetic Association* says you can predict your future weight based on what you are eating today. Boston University researchers analysed the dietary habits of more than 700 women to determine who became overweight over a 12-year period. Those who routinely ate more servings of nutrient-dense fruits and vegetables and other lean foods were the least likely to become overweight.

This illustrates that we need to pay attention to our overall diet and eating patterns as early as possible if we are to manage our weight over the long term.

YOUNG, FREE AND SINGLE DAS MANAGEMENT

'I feel too exhausted to exercise when it's the time of the month'

Don't panic if you can't drag yourself through a workout during your period. Your hormone levels change as you go through your monthly cycle, and these have a direct impact on your energy levels.

Preliminary research also indicates that your ability to burn fat varies at different times in your monthly cycle. Scientists asked a small group of women with normal menstrual cycles to do a single rigorous cycling workout 5–7 days after the start of their periods and again 5–7 days after ovulation (usually around day 14). The women not only felt more sluggish early in their cycles, but they also burned less fat when they exercised at this time. When oestrogen and progesterone levels are low, as happens early in your cycle, your body burns more carbohydrate during exercise, which creates more metabolic waste and makes exercise feel harder. So instead of pushing yourself through a tough workout during your period, plan your workouts around your menstrual cycle. Opt for yoga, Pilates, or simple strength and toning exercises during your period and more high intensity cardiovascular work-outs during the second half of your cycle.

Yes, calorie expenditure is still important but this way you will be instilling the habit of taking regular exercise – plus you'll be adding variety to your training schedule and hence challenging a wider set of muscle groups.

Get in the mood

Accepting that exercise and physical activity are important in keeping that size off is one thing, but summoning the motivation to do it is quite another – particularly when hormonal highs and lows come into the equation. I have noticed many of my clients want to skip their workout when their mood isn't ideal. It's almost as if they don't have the mental energy to switch gears. However, the trick lies in finding the right workout to match the mood you're in. Some workouts have a calming effect while others are stimulating.

So rather than let an 'off' mood stop you exercising, harness it by doing the type of exercise that feels right. This will help you feel more confident about how you can fit physical activity into your life, even when life is challenging and your willpower is low. You will find plenty of ideas on how to choose exercise according to your mood in the table on pages 276–278.

EXERCISE TO BOOST YOUR MOOD

You are	You need	Suggestions
Feeling low	Mild exercise of moderate intensity. Studies show that even exercising at 40% of your maximum heart rate can lift your mood.	Ditch the high-energy stuff and opt for more leisurely activities: cycle, do some gardening or take a brisk walk in the park. View your exercise as mental relaxation and rejuvenation rather than purely physical exercise.
Feeling bored	Exercise that gets you mingling with other people is an easy way to beat boredom. Team sports are a great option.	Try tennis, or golf or enrol in a skills-improvement class. Go for a bike ride on a regular basis. Being outside with other people is invigorating and engages your mind. Plan a run with your girlfriends to catch up on gossip, rather than going to the pub.

You are	You need	Suggestions
Feeling angry	As tempting as it may sound, taking your anger out in a kickboxing class is not the best option. Many experts maintain that aggressive activities fuel anger rather than diffuse it. Instead, employ diversion tactics and do something that stops you mulling over whatever is making you angry.	Try a new sport or an exercise class at the gym that you've not tried before. Learning new moves will focus your mind away from what has been upsetting you.
Stressed-out	When your brain is fit to burst with all the things on your 'to do' list, you need to create some quiet space and do something that doesn't involve much concentration. This will allow your brain to quieten and will give you a breathing space.	Repetitive movements are ideal, such as swimming, cycling, jogging or walking. These activities require little mental input and can reduce feelings of stress and induce calmness.

You are	You need	Suggestions
On cloud nine	Being in a good mood can derail your good intentions and the effectiveness of a workout as much as a bad mood. Take advantage of your confident and upbeat mood and go out and challenge yourself.	Why not try to run 1 mile more than usual, set yourself a new strength training routine, or try a new workout video. Use that positivity to help you step outside your comfort zone – it'll give you more workout options for the future.

'I can't stop munching just before my period!'

Just before your period begins, your metabolic rate increases, which means you are actually burning more calories. The problem is, this genuine increase in metabolic rate makes you feel hungrier and this is compounded by an increased demand for magnesium, which can cause you to crave sweet foods. In reality, the body only uses an additional 120–150 calories a day at this time, so when we reach for a chocolate bar we're taking on double the number of extra calories that the body actually needs. Check out page 194 for a wide range of 100-calorie snack ideas that will satisfy your cravings without overcompensating. Also ensure you are getting sufficient magnesium in your diet. The recommended daily allowance is 300mg. The table below gives some rich sources.

MAGNESIUM FOOD TABLE

Food	Magnesium Content
40g Bran Flakes with 150ml skimmed milk	70mg
2 slices wholemeal bread	58mg
1 medium-sized jacket potato	60mg
200g baked beans	60mg
1 banana	34mg
50g pack of mixed nuts and raisins	65mg
180g cooked brown rice	77mg
6 dried apricots	20mg
25g plain chocolate	25mg

'I feel moody and crave comfort food at certain times of the month'
There's a growing body of evidence that suggests specific foods have an effect on our mood. Some foods make us feel content and satiated, while others make us feel more alert. Eating to beat your mood swings is a great way of navigating those monthly highs and lows. Check out the Eat to Boost Your Mood table on the following pages for some guidance.

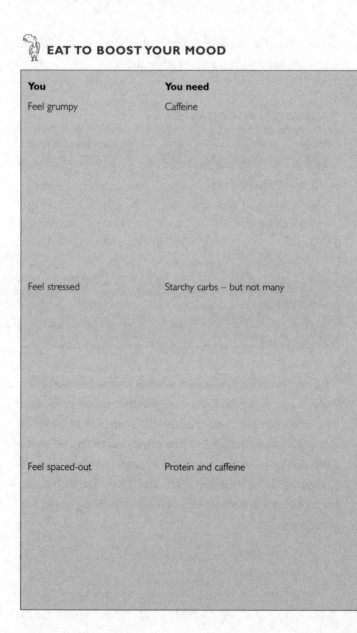

🍴 EAT TO BOOST YOUR MOOD

You	You need
Feel grumpy	Caffeine
Feel stressed	Starchy carbs – but not many
Feel spaced-out	Protein and caffeine

Why?

Caffeine is a mood elevator. A cup of coffee stimulates the receptor sites in the brain to become more active. Despite persistent anti-caffeine rumblings, the overwhelming evidence is that a *moderate* amount is not harmful to most women. However, a coffee or cola habit can wreak havoc on the emotions of some people (in some women as little as two cups of coffee a day has this effect). If you've noticed loop-the-loop emotions and think you might be particularly sensitive, try to quit; if you find you feel better, then a few cups are probably not doing you any harm.

Starchy carbohydrates stimulate the release of serotonin, a mood-regulating brain transmitter, into the bloodstream, which makes us feel calm and lethargic. So bagels, jams, mashed potato and other comfort foods are popular natural choices when you feel stressed. However, these comfort foods can be calorie dense and of low nutrient value – plus there's a tendency to overeat when stressed anyway. So go easy on them. More than 1,000 calories of anything in a single sitting will leave you sleepy and inattentive, making you even less likely to move and expend those calories.

Eating an adequate amount of protein will help keep your energy level even, especially if you are prone to eating too many carbs. During digestion, protein breaks down into amino acid building blocks, which will pump up the production of neurotransmitters (dopamine, norepinephrine and epinephrine) that can make you feel more alert. Caffeine, of course, has been demonstrated to increase alertness and pairing your coffee with a meal containing lean protein can help.

You	You need
Feel tired	Water – followed by a little starch and a larger bit of protein
Feel 'PMSy'	Calcium and low-fat dairy and magnesium-rich foods

Why?

The first symptom of dehydration is fatigue. Even mild dehydration can make you feel worn out and lethargic because it causes a dip in blood volume and it is blood that carries oxygen to the brain and body. When the transport of oxygen isn't efficient your body doesn't get signals to your various bodily systems as quickly. The recommendation from the British Dietetic Association is 5 pints a day – three in the form of water and the remaining two from water-packed vegetables and soups. A 1 per cent decrease in your hydration levels can bring about a 10 per cent decrease in performance – so think water first! Carbohydrate paired with protein will give you lasting energy. Stay away from biscuits or sweets and make your carbohydrate source fruit. High-fibre fruits won't cause insulin levels to peak, as sweets do, and will help you feel full for longer.

If you are moody and suffer cramps each month, pack your diet with calcium from low-fat dairy foods and supplements. Researchers found that women who were given 1,200 milligrams of calcium carbonate daily had almost a 50 per cent reduction in PMS symptoms after three cycles. Seventy three per cent of women who took 1,000 milligrams of calcium daily for three months reported fewer emotional swings and less irritability.

'Period pain stops me exercising'

Hormone-like chemicals called prostaglandins are to blame for menstrual cramps, as they make nerves more sensitive and intensify our experience of pain. If you are very susceptible to period pain, you may be very sensitive to prostaglandins, or your body may simply produce more of them. Menstrual cramps (uterine muscle contractions caused by the elevated release of prostaglandins) tend to be stronger and more frequent during the first two days of your period, so this is when you are most likely to feel like skipping a workout.

While you should always listen to your body, there are some strategies worth trying to reduce the pain of menstrual cramps – and one of those is, you guessed it, exercise! In fact, in a recent study carried out in Australia, women who were highly active reported less period pain and PMS symptoms than sedentary women.

Here are some tips for getting through the monthly grind …

- **Take pain medication**

  The best painkillers for period pain are ibuprofen and naproxen sodium. These are both non-steroidal anti-inflammatory drugs that reduce prostaglandin production. For best results, take at the first sign of period pain and for the first day or two of your period. Naproxen sodium is best taken every 8–12 hours: ibuprofen every 4–6 hours. (If you have teenage daughters suffering from

period pain, a naproxen sodium-based drug is probably
most appropriate as they can take one before they go to
school and one on return). Both these drugs are available
over the counter, but if they don't work speak to your
doctor about stronger versions. Birth control pills also
help reduce menstrual cramps and heavy bleeding.

- **Apply heat**
  One of the oldest remedies – heat – now comes in
  portable 'heat packs', which you wear against your body
  under your clothes. The heat helps the muscles relax and
  acts as an analgesic, increasing blood flow to the tissues,
  which is thought to help dilute prostaglandins. A good old
  hot water bottle works just as well at night.

- **Don't skimp on exercise**
  Exercise increases blood flow and can help relieve the
  muscle tension that contributes to cramps. The endorphins
  released in response to exercise can also help mask pain.
  You may not want to exercise as vigorously, but moderate
  physical activity will help.

- **Check your calcium intake**
  Studies have shown women who take 1200mg of calcium
  get significant relief from PMS symptoms, including painful
  cramps. The recommended daily amount in the UK is
  800mg for pre-menopausal women. Here are some of the
  best sources:

Skimmed milk (200ml glass)	250mg
Cheddar (1 slice 20g)	160mg
Canned pink salmon (with bones 100g)	310mg
Canned sardines (100g)	380mg
Steamed spinach (1 cup)	170mg
Natural yoghurt (200g carton)	420mg
Tofu (100g)	130mg
Chickpeas (100g)	160mg
Dried figs (50g)	115mg
So Good (soya milk, 200ml glass)	220mg

- **Acupuncture**
  Acupuncture has been highly effective for pain relief in
  post-operative patients so there is no reason why it could
  not be beneficial for painful periods, too.
- **Top up your omega-3 fatty acids**
  Foods that are high in omega-3 fatty acids, such as oily fish,
  walnuts, flaxseed and dark green leafy vegetables, reduce
  the body's production of prostaglandins and hence the
  severity of period pains.

If the pain you are experiencing is still severe, despite
having tried these approaches, speak to your doctor, as
it could be a sign of endometriosis, fibroids, a sexually-
transmitted disease, or pelvic inflammatory disease.

Case Study: Sarah's Success

'I had read that diet could affect your period, and specifically period pain, but I really didn't have any idea how much until I became a lot more diligent about eating oily fish. I now make a concerted effort to eat oily fish at least four times a week in the fortnight leading up to my period. It sounds strange but it has made a huge difference to me. Just how effective it is was made clear to me recently, when I let my DAS management slip due to the turmoil of moving house. I noticed I had far worse period cramps, which made me less inclined to exercise. So for me eating oily fish has two benefits: I experience less period pain plus I'm much more motivated to exercise instead of grabbing a chocolate bar.'

'The pill is making me fat'

There are many different types of contraceptive pill on the market. These are generally a combination of oestrogen and progesterone or progesterone only (also known as the mini pill). The combined pill tends to have the most impact on some women's weight, because oestrogen can contribute to fluid retention or cause an increase in appetite. However, your response to whatever pill you are on will be individual, dependent upon your metabolic rate and hormone sensitivity. If you are concerned that your pill may be contributing to you gaining a size, speak to your doctor about changing to either a low dose pill (although bear in mind that though it may be more suitable in terms of weight management, it may be less suitable in other ways), or the mini pill.

But whatever you do, remember you are in control – try to avoid blaming all your weight issues on the pill, as it is likely to play only a small part in your size.

'I don't have time to cook'
You may have big ideas and big plans for your future, but don't let your lifestyle get in the way of looking after yourself! A busy career and social life may leave you short of time and you probably find yourself lacking the energy to exercise and eat healthily, so here are some tips:

• **Find your workout wedge**
You don't need a whole hour to work out; instead, find your workout wedge. Your workout wedge is the time you can find in your day to fit in exercise. Ideally, this should be 30 minutes of continuous exercise but let's be realistic – that's not always possible. Look back at section two to find lots of different workout wedges to suit your body and the amount of time you have available. To fit in your workout wedge you need to be a little creative with how you make time. You could perhaps fit it in during your lunch break, or when you have completed a report and you're waiting for a response. Alternatively, many of my clients have found they can fit in a workout wedge when they're waiting for their dinner to cook. See page 148 for 'dinner and a workout wedge' ideas.

- **Eat to boost your energy, not bust your belt**

  Little and often is the way to go to sustain constant energy levels. Skipping two meals then having a huge dinner will leave you feeling bloated and devoid of energy. If you follow the meal suggestions in section two you'll have the right balance of proteins and carbohydrate to fuel your demanding schedule.

'I end up binge eating after a few too many drinks'

Not only is alcohol laden with calories, it also lowers our resistance to overeating and deludes us into thinking we're starving. That's why a few drinks after work often results in us going home, not with a hunky man, but with a bag of chips or a kebab! And this, of course, only adds to the substantial amount of calories you've already taken on board with all those Bacardi Breezers or glasses of Chardonnay.

One of the key defences against alcohol-induced bingeing is to eat before you go out. If you're at work, a small snack, such as a couple of rice cakes spread with peanut butter, is easy to prepare (see 100-calorie snack ideas on page 194 for more inspiration). If you're at home, check out the Five-Minute Carb Curfew Meals on page 231 for quick nutritious recipes that won't eat into your social life. Another way of combating the problem is to ensure you are well hydrated. If you know it's going to be a big night, then drink lots of water throughout the day and slip in a glass of sparkling water or another soft drink between each alcoholic one. Not only will you survive the evening much better, you're also more likely to wake up without a hangover the following day – and stick to your exercise schedule.

Case study: Jessica's Story

Jessica's social life was important to her and she often went for a drink after work. However, as she approached her thirties she found her dress size getting a bit on the large side. She knew she was drinking too much – and that stuffing herself at Ali Baba's kebab shop on the way home wasn't helping matters! Her answer? Whenever she went out with her friends straight from work she would pre-book a particular train home. This way she knew she had to make that train, or miss it and pay another fare. This meant Jessica was leaving the pub a little earlier – when she still had enough willpower to pass Ali Baba's – and could then enjoy a more nutritious meal when she got home. The upshot was she lost 6 pounds without too much hardship and without missing out on her social life. The only one who missed out was Ali Baba – or rather his purse!

🍷 YOU ARE ... SETTLING DOWN

For most of us, there eventually comes a time when evenings cuddled up on the sofa seem more appealing than a night on the town. Meeting Mr Right becomes more important than having fun with the latest Mr 'Wrong-but-Fun'. Our social lives become less frenetic and we begin to think about setting up home, finding a partner, perhaps getting married and starting a family. While fewer hangovers and late-night kebab shop raids are a good thing, when it comes to health and weight management, the nesting instinct can bring its own set of challenges. Let's look at some of the key challenges that women entering the 'nesting phase' have to contend with ...

SETTLING DOWN DAS MANAGEMENT

'I'm moving in with my partner'
Moving in with your loved one is one of life's great pleasures – but it can also be dangerous ground as far as your weight goes. Women often gain 10 pounds when they marry or move in with their partner. It's a combination of being 'settled' and simply eating more. Men can eat more than women without gaining weight and you don't need to be a newlywed to find yourself mimicking your partner's eating habits. Sharing food and drink in a relaxed social way is an important part of your intimate

relationship – but first, learn how to handle these DAS saboteurs …

- **He brings home fast food and goodies**
  Take a trip to the supermarket together and point out what you really like, as you put things in the trolley together. That way, when he goes to the supermarket solo he picks up things that go to your heart and not your hips! And if he must have crisps and chocolate, ask him to keep them out of sight.
- **You start eating the same portion sizes**
  A woman roughly needs about a third fewer calories than a man, so when you start absentmindedly serving yourself the same amount as him – STOP right there! Try these tips:
  1 Downsize your plate – give him a dinner plate while you have a large side plate or salad plate.
  2 Let him get a head start – this will prevent you finishing first and going to get seconds simply because he's still eating. Sip your drink or nibble some crudités before you start.
  3 Leave what you don't need – if he consistently serves you large portions or one the same size as his, try to leave a third on your plate. Do this regularly enough and he'll soon get the message and serve you less.
- **He cooks fattening foods**
  This can be a tricky one and depends on your partner's personality. Try these tips to see how you get on:

1   Tell him you love his cooking but, every now and again, suggest a less fattening recipe.

2   Tell him that his cooking is great but eating all that fattening food is reducing your sex drive and you have some great ideas to boost bedroom activity! I have found that this one normally works with newly-hitched clients!

Case study: Jane's Story

Jane met and then moved in with a really gorgeous guy. She was a fit girl who had always been careful about her diet. Gorgeous guy, however, was one of these annoying creatures who looks like a Greek god but eats like a Trojan. He was also Italian, which meant molto pasta was the order of the day! So Jane had her work cut out. After three months she found she had gained 4 pounds and was feeling less confident about herself physically and this, she felt, was affecting her sex life. However, she wanted to carry on enjoying her sex life so she tried the fattening-food-reduces-your-sex-drive argument and found it worked – now her gorgeous guy is a Carb Curfew advocate, too!

'I've lost my confidence'

While becoming part of a couple can be wonderful, it can also leave you with a feeling of being 'half' the person you once were. It's common for couples who move in togeth-er to go out less than they did when they were single or courting, so there's less exposure to confidence-boosting interaction with other people. Women are also notoriously good at putting their needs at the bottom of the list. You may find that ironing your partner's shirts, or entertaining his family, takes up the time you would otherwise have spent working out or on some other hobby. This can have a knock-on effect on your diet, as you tend to put your new partner's needs before your own – perhaps serving far heavier evening meals that please him but aren't really your cup of tea. Revisit step 6 in section one to remind yourself of how to get up on that pedestal. Successful relationships are about balance and it's important that your own needs are being met if you are to maintain your self-esteem and find the time and energy to devote to your drop a size action plan.

'I'm pregnant'

This is one time when gaining a size (or two) is positively essential! See page 302 for the DAS pregnancy management plan to find out how to have a fit, healthy and happy pregnancy and page 309 for ideas on shifting that post-baby fat.

'My relationship has broken down'

Getting dumped can actually be one of the quickest ways to drop a size, as a broken heart often triggers a lack of hunger. However, in the long term, feelings of loss and chronic stress often result in people gradually eating more or drinking more alcohol, leading to a gradual increase in weight. To counteract this and move on, take the following steps:

- **Focus on something other than your loss.**
  Try taking up a new hobby or activity to help you stay busy. Successful activities girlfriends of mine have tried are yoga, singing lessons, a wine course, learning a language and upholstery evening classes.
- **Acknowledge the hurt, but move on.**
  Clear away all the lovey-dovey pictures and replace them with pictures of friends who give you love in a different way. We have already seen how self-esteem is the foundation to your successful weight and health goals, rather than a product of it, so look back at steps 2 and 3 in section one. Relearning how to value yourself and do what you can, right now, will help you live in and enjoy the moment, rather than dwelling on the past or worrying about the future.
- **Do all of the above willingly!**
  I know this sounds strange, but actually wanting to do all of these things, rather than going through the motions, will help you heal quicker and put you back in control.

WARNING SIGNS – THE CHILD-BEARING YEARS

You ...	Warning sign
Move in with your partner	Your partner's needs can start to become far more important than yours and you fall lower and lower down your priority list.
Don't get promoted at work and a colleague gets promoted above you	Your confidence is knocked and this starts to eat away at your self-esteem, which has a knock-on effect in other parts of your life. You stop remembering other successes and achievements in your life and how you have the ability to positively affect the course of your life.
Want to get in shape quickly for that Greek holiday with your mates	You have left it to the 11th hour again to squeeze into that bikini. You need results and you need them fast. You curse yourself for leaving it to the last minute again.
Become a new mum	You are exhausted and are constantly trying to juggle things to provide for new baby, new changes in the home – let alone trying to convince your partner he is still having a relationship with a sex goddess!

Action

Get yourself back on that pedestal! Re-visit step 6 in section one. Successful relationships are about balance and while us females tend to want to make everything run smoothly, this does not mean we have to start sowing the seeds of self-neglect!

Start making friends with yourself again. Re-visit steps 1, 2 and 3 in section one. You need to get that brain under control again and make sure what you say, what you do and what you think are all going in the same direction. Don't let your negative thoughts hinder your efforts or affect how you feel about yourself.

So you've found your small G spot again! It's about time you started to find a larger G spot and enjoyed the benefits for longer. Re-visit step 7 in section one and find that large G spot. You may also find it useful to look at step 5 on establishing the here and now. Getting in shape does not have to involve pressing the stop button, it's more a case of putting together a series of 'now' moments.

Don't panic about being a juggler, try to learn a new mantra — what will be will be. Re-visit steps 5 and 6 in section one to put things in perspective. This is a very delicate time when your hormones can be challenging your self-esteem. Focus on small actions and carving just 5 minutes for yourself each day.

Guys need guidance too!

Don't think it's any easier for a man to get away with fast food and no exercise. Chilling new research published in the *Journal of the American Medical Association* shows that being obese (at least 30–40 pounds overweight) at the age of 30 can cut up to 6 years off a man's life expectancy. Obesity at 20 years of age can cut it by up to 20 years. So if your man is a little too cuddly, check out the fundamentals in section two and get him back on track. Many of my male clients find my Carb Curfew a really simple weight loss strategy that delivers real benefits.

Case study: David's Success

David was a GP who loved his food, his social life and his wine. However, his lifestyle was starting to take its toll on his physique. He embarked on my weight management course and lost 28 pounds in 10 weeks. Two years later he has still kept the weight off. Despite holidaying in Italy, David also finds that he now only gains about 3 pounds from his holiday excesses and, once he gets back on the Carb Curfew, it drops off really quickly.

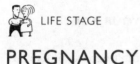 LIFE STAGE

PREGNANCY

Being pregnant is the greatest life-changing experience a woman can have. Nothing – including your body – will ever be the same again. Women's mental and physical experiences of the nine-month miracle differ greatly, but there's no doubt that pregnancy is going to impact on your energy levels and your eating and exercise patterns. It's also likely to have an influence on how you feel about yourself, which can have a knock-on effect on your behaviour. While pregnancy is a time when you must put the needs of your growing baby first, it doesn't mean you should neglect your own needs. In fact, sticking to a healthy eating plan and incorporating regular, safe exercise into your routine is as good for your baby as it is for you.

Does this tickle your G spot?
Women who are physically active before and after giving birth tend to feel happier and adapt better to being a mother. They also tend to have a better experience of labour and delivery, and are more confident about being a mum.

WHAT'S HAPPENING INSIDE YOUR BODY

Well, this is one time when you can't expect to maintain your size. The general UK guideline is that you should put on around 20 lbs during pregnancy. Guidelines by the US Institute of Medicine are more specific: they recommend 25–35 lbs of weight gain for normal weight women, 15 lbs for obese women and 28–40 lbs for underweight women during a full-term pregnancy.

Half of the extra weight is made up of the foetus itself, plus the uterus and its contents – the rest is as a result of increased body fat and fluid, including the breast tissue. The majority of the weight gained is stored at the front of the body, which alters your centre of gravity. In order to compensate, the pelvis tilts forward and the curve in the lower back increases – it is this that causes the lower back-ache that affects 50 per cent of pregnant women.

Physiologically speaking, the effects of pregnancy are remarkably similar to those of endurance exercise (which is why some people refer to it as nine months in training!). During the first trimester, blood pressure generally tends to drop, but it returns to normal in the 2nd and 3rd trimesters. Blood volume increases by as much as 40–50 per cent and the amount of blood pumped out per beat of the heart also goes up, though in the final trimester it begins to decline again, which – given the increased blood volume – can cause blood to pool in the limbs, leading to varicose veins.

Even though blood volume increases, the amount of red blood cells stays the same. The red blood cells are responsible for carrying energy-giving oxygen to the muscles. So the extra blood volume actually dilutes the concentration of available red blood cells. This creates a feeling of greater fatigue, which many pregnant women will be all too familiar with. In addition, the resting heart rate rises by 15–20 bpm, which will make exercise harder work. The increased levels of progesterone can also increase ventilation, so that breathing is quicker and deeper.

Some of the more laborious side effects of pregnancy include an increase in digestion 'transit' time, resulting in constipation and indigestion, fluid retention and skin irritation. In addition, higher volumes of urine production, coupled with the increasingly heavy uterus pressing down on the bladder, can make you feel you need to pee constantly. However, despite all the discomforts of pregnancy, research shows it is not a time to permanently put your feet up. In fact, regular exercise is associated with fewer occurrences of these classic pregnancy discomforts. So don't be put off.

BENEFITS OF AN ACTIVE PREGNANCY

- According to a study by the University of Michigan School of Nursing, moderate exercise during pregnancy lowered blood pressure and reduced the risk of developing gestational hypertension. (The women in the study exercised for 30 minutes, three times a week.)

- Women who engage in regular exercise experience easier labour and tend to have their babies on time.
- Women who exercise tend to have higher birth weight babies.
- Exercise during pregnancy seems to reduce pregnancy-related discomforts such as nausea and fatigue.
- Women who exercise through pregnancy gain less weight than sedentary women during their term.

Does this tickle your G spot?

Although pregnant women are commonly said to be 'eating for two', gaining more than is necessary (see guidelines above) puts you at six times the risk of being obese by your child's first birthday. The extra pounds also increase the risk of high blood pressure, heart disease and diabetes. So don't think of yourself as eating for two – yes your calorie needs do increase but you only require an additional 200 calories a day.

PREGNANCY DAS MANAGEMENT PLAN

'Is it safe to exercise while pregnant?'
The answer is most definitely YES! Recent guidelines recommend that in the absence of medical complications, pregnant women should engage in 30 minutes or more of moderate intensity exercise on most, if not all, days of the

week. So if you are already active, don't let pregnancy cramp your style. If you're not active, then get moving – but take it slowly and carefully. A hormone called relaxin is secreted during pregnancy and this, along with an increase in progesterone, has the effect of softening the body's ligaments (particularly those around the back and pelvis) in preparation for delivery. Therefore, later on in pregnancy, the instability of the joints caused by ligament laxity can make weight-bearing exercise, such as running or aerobics, risky, as you are more susceptible to musculoskeletal injuries.

'What sort of exercise is appropriate?'
Ideal activities include brisk walking, swimming, biking, low impact aerobics, jogging (if you were a runner *before* you became pregnant) and even low to moderate intensity strength training. Avoid contact sports, as well as activities with an increased risk of falling, such as skiing. Don't go scuba diving either, as it would put the foetus at risk from decompression sickness.

TIPS FOR EXERCISING SAFELY WHILE PREGNANT
- Avoid getting overheated – don't exercise in hot or humid conditions.
- Stop your workout if you have any pain, dizziness, increased shortness of breath, chest pain, muscle weakness, premature labour, vaginal bleeding, irregular or rapid heartbeat.

- Never exercise to the point of exhaustion.
- Drink enough water so that you are hydrated before, during and after your workout.
- Reduce the intensity of your workouts and put your pre-pregnancy fitness goals to one side temporarily.
- Don't overstrain joints, which are more susceptible to injury now, due to the ligament-softening hormone relaxin.
- After the first trimester, avoid motionless standing positions, such as those found in yoga, or lying back during exercise, as these reduce blood flow to the placenta.
- Listen to your body at all times.

'I have no energy'

Carrying all that extra weight around alone could sap your energy, but all the other physiological changes associated with pregnancy also come into play and this combination of factors can make healthy lifestyle choices seem like too much effort. Try the following strategies:

- **Accept help**
  When others offer help or say 'is there anything I can do?', say yes! One client of mine, who had a particularly tough pregnancy, got her friends and family to help stock up her freezer with homemade soups, stews and other dishes that she could just put in the oven. This meant she could maintain a healthy diet without having to traipse to the supermarket.

- **Opt for convenience**

  You might normally think buying ready-peeled veg or pre-washed salad an unnecessary indulgence, but if that's what it takes to get you eating healthily, then do it. This is a time when ensuring you get your five-a-day is really important, so think about canned fruit or fruit from the fresh fruit bar, frozen vegetables and bottled juices and smoothies.

- **Don't be hard on yourself**

  If you really can't get out of the chair, give yourself a break. There's no point giving yourself a hard time for not making it to the gym three times a week. Remember step 5 in section one – you might not be able to do everything right, but do what you can, right now. It may simply mean some gentle stretching, a 10-minute walk, or a session at the pool that involves more floating than swimming.

Does this tickle your G spot?

Why not drop those extra pounds before you get pregnant? Being overweight while carrying your baby increases your risk of gestational diabetes, pre-eclampsia and having a non-elective Caesarean delivery.

'I feel too sick to eat properly or exercise'
Morning sickness is enough to put even the most motivated woman off-track as far as exercise and healthy eating are concerned. Morning sickness is caused by high levels of a hormone called HCG. The good news is, it rarely lasts beyond the first three months of pregnancy. These tips may help:

- Have small frequent snacks, as these are easier to tolerate than larger meals.
- If you are usually a morning exerciser, try switching your workout time to afternoon or evening when the nausea has abated.
- Try drinking ginger tea, which has been shown to reduce feelings of nausea.

Ginger Tea
Peel a 2cm piece of fresh ginger, place in a teapot and pour over boiling water. Leave for 5 minutes for the flavours to infuse and then drink.

'I feel too self-conscious or intimidated to exercise'
If you feel self-conscious about your bump, then you could always work out at home, or in your back garden. If you're worried about being challenged about exercising 'in your condition' – don't be. Few people would say

anything and if they do it's only those who are complete-ly out of touch with modern thinking on pregnancy and exercise. Such people don't realize that you are doing both yourself and your growing baby a favour by being active, and that you're not putting the foetus at risk. If you get heckled, ignore it and if someone asks you about it, then put them in the picture!

'Exercise is uncomfortable'
Many women feel uncomfortable in the abdominal region during pregnancy, as the ligaments supporting the uterus stretch and movement can tug at them. Maternity knick-ers that go over the bump, rather than under it, offer more support for when you are being active. Other women use maternity belts, swimsuits or cycling shorts to reduce movement and add support to the area. If it's your boobs that feel uncomfortable during activity, ensure you are wearing a well-fitting sports bra – or even two. Remember, you'll need a different size bra than before you were pregnant.

'I am eating for two'
The increase in levels of progesterone during pregnancy does stimulate appetite, and yes, it's true, you do need more calories when you are pregnant. However, as I men-tioned earlier, you only need an extra 200 calories a day – so that in no way gives you carte blanche to eat everything in sight! Try to maintain the principles of healthy eating

that you learned about in section two, but simply increase your portion sizes a little. Also ensure that you are not mistaking thirst for hunger – make sure you are well hydrated.

Many of the women who view pregnancy as one of the few times in life when they can eat whatever they like are those who are stuck with considerable amounts of excess weight to shift after the baby's been born.

RECLAIMING YOUR BODY
AFTER PREGNANCY

So you are a proud mum with a beautiful baby – but all too often, that is not what you think or see. Being a new mum is fraught with emotions – not just because of surging hormones but also because it's all new territory, and territory that has to be explored under conditions of very little time, energy or sleep. Four out of five women experience some form of 'baby blues' in the first fortnight after giving birth. In addition, many new mums report that while they may have been very large in their third trimester, at least their body was firm and toned. And now, well, jelly belly has come to town in a BIG way!

But don't lose heart; be positive – you can lose that post-baby weight. Researchers have found that the more positive feelings a woman has about motherhood, the more likely she is to exercise frequently after giving birth. A word of advice: it is widely acknowledged that post birth you should not do any rigorous exercise until you have had your post-natal check-up. For a normal birth this is carried out after six weeks and for a C section, at week eleven.

Reclaiming your body is all about becoming aware of your body as it is now. You will need to re-establish the connection between your brain and your body and retrain the muscles that have become distended as your baby grew inside you. This awareness is necessary before you can successfully shift that post-baby fat. So successful DAS management is not all about getting back into the gym. Yes, you're going to have to put some effort in, but a few exercises, with time invested wisely for your body and your head, can reap rewards without you struggling to find the time or the energy. Remember, it took nine months for you to gain all the baby weight so it's okay for you to take a little while to lose it.

WHAT'S HAPPENING INSIDE YOUR BODY

Post-baby, your hormones are having a field day. Hormones that were soaring during your pregnancy now plummet, which can leave you feeling melancholic, stressed or irritable. A woman is thought to be more prone to post-natal depression if she has suffered badly from PMS, depression during the pregnancy or if it is a first baby.

Two of the hormones that contribute to the general mêlée are prolactin and oxytocin. Prolactin is a hormone that stimulates breast tissue to produce milk; it also rises in response to any kind of stress. Oxytocin is the 'bonding' hormone, which is released during labour – it is thought to help facilitate the bond between mother and baby and between adult partners. Interestingly, oxytocin is also released during orgasm, possibly to encourage the two participating parties to stay together and bring up baby!

DAS MANAGEMENT PLAN FOR RECLAIMING YOUR BODY

Reclaiming your ideal size after having a baby is one of the biggest weight management challenges. The problems are threefold: your body has changed physiologically, you have a major time and energy commitment that you didn't have before and, finally, your mental state may have changed so that you feel your size is no longer the big issue it was before. Here are some of the common obstacles that women face in this challenging time – and some suggestions and tips.

'I'm worried exercise will jeopardize my breast-feeding!'
Moderate intensity exercise will not affect your breast milk. Studies have shown that aerobic exercise, such as brisk walking, swimming and dancing, while breast-feeding will not affect the quantity or composition of breast milk, or the weight of your baby.

Encouraging research from the University of North Carolina suggests that breastfeeding mothers who are overweight can lose weight through a sensible diet and exercise program without fear of harming their child. Women with a BMI of 25–30 (see page 7 to assess your BMI) cut calories by 500 per day and did 15 minutes aerobic exercise, adding 2 minutes a day, up to 45 minutes after 10 weeks. They lost an average of 10 pounds at the end of 10 weeks and milk production and infant contentment were not affected. The researchers warn, however, that breastfeeding mothers who are only 5 pounds overweight should delay losing weight, as a low calorie intake may affect milk production.

Does this tickle your G spot?

Those who have not returned to their pre-pregnancy weight after about six months will most likely retain the extra weight. So be patient but firm with yourself – and those around you – as this is a crucial time for your DAS management.

'*I eat because I'm bored and depressed*'

In a recent survey on food and feelings, it was found that 53 per cent of respondents overate when they were bored, 30 per cent turned to food when they were sad and only nine per cent reached for food when happy. So you're not alone.

The first months after the birth are undoubtedly very trying. Your days of partying seem a lifetime ago and romantic candlelit suppers for two are rapidly replaced by takeaways, nappy bags and nights in front of the TV; while nights of hot passion are replaced by games of spoof for whose turn it is to see to the baby in the middle of the night. These factors, plus that fact that you get out less and potentially lose your sense of identity, can impact on your self-esteem. You may want to reclaim your body, but often your hormones are raging, sending you on an emotional roller coaster of euphoria and self-doubt.

First, get the support of others – whether that means joining a mother and toddler group, getting your mother or sister round more often, or meeting up with your old friends from work. Don't shut yourself away and take comfort in the biscuit tin. Recent research found that women suffering from moderate depression or anxiety ate an average of 118 extra calories each day. They also ate fewer fruit and veg. If your post-baby blues carry on for a year, that could translate to a gain of 12 pounds in one year – that's more than the average baby's birth weight!

Try to trade one high calorie snack for low calorie carrot sticks or an apple every day. Stock up on frozen, canned and pre-packed veg as well as frozen fruits, thus avoiding the problem of never having any veg around. Ask visitors and family to bring you healthy groceries as opposed to sweet things and cakes. Okay, so your local coffee shop doesn't sell carrot sticks but you can still choose the healthiest thing on the menu.

WARNING SIGNS – RECLAIMING YOUR BODY

You...	Warning sign
It's only post-baby fat and it will drop off as soon as I stop feeding	Well yes, it may well do – but in practice becoming physically active as soon as possible and taking control of your eating will have the greatest impact on your size. Studies have shown that when you stop breast-feeding the final five pounds do start to drop off, but many people have a lot more than five pounds of body fat to lose!
My partner loves me the way I am	Well yes, he does and that's great – but how about you loving yourself and having the pride to keep yourself fit and healthy for your growing family. As your child grows you will become an important role model for them in the way you live your life; the way you eat and exercise. No one wants to wish ill health upon their own child so if you find it hard to get enough motivation for yourself, think of your future family and use that as a small stepping stone to get you going.

Action

Look at section one, step 5. You need to address these issues here and now. Waiting six months until you stop breast-feeding will only make the task harder. Have a read and get going girl!

You need to re-visit section one, step 7 to find your G spot and find it fast! To start with, make a list of small motivations and then put them all together to gain momentum to hit that big G spot.

WARNING SIGNS – RECLAIMING YOUR BODY

You...	Warning sign
I'm going to get pregnant again soon so I don't need to bother losing the weight until I've finished having my kids	You know you want a big family and so you may as well try to have them all in one bout! Well this may make sense – but you will be able to conceive more easily and have a healthier pregnancy if you're a healthy weight. Studies have shown that not losing your pregnancy baby weight within six months makes it extra hard to shift. In addition, getting your life back on track is an important part of giving yourself some time and not falling to the bottom of your priority list.
Are a new mum	You are exhausted and are constantly trying to juggle things to provide for new baby, new changes in the home – let alone trying to convince your partner he is still having a relationship with a sex goddess!

Action

Get a grip – you don't need to carve your body into that of a supermodel but do make some investments for you and your health. Re-visit section one, step 2 about making friends with yourself in the mirror. This will help stay focussed on your body and should prevent things getting too out of hand.

Don't panic about being a juggler, try to learn a new mantra – what will be will be. Re-visit section one, steps 5 and 6 to put things into perspective. This is a very delicate time when your hormones, lack of sleep and new life challenges can affect your self-esteem. Focus on small actions and carving out just 5 minutes for yourself each day.

'I get painful boobs when I exercise'
The golden rule is, feed first, then exercise later to reduce the discomfort of full and heavy breasts. A good sports bra is also essential – styles that encapsulate rather than compress the breasts are preferable when you are breastfeeding. Some women prefer to wear two bras at the same time for added support and security. If your breasts ache at the mere thought of aerobic exercise, you can still take positive action by working on reclaiming your deep abdominal muscles. See section two page 136 for a waist-whittling workout wedge.

'I have no support from my partner when it comes to getting back in shape'
Just as you have experienced tremendous change, so too has your partner – so don't be surprised if you don't get the level of support you expected. The changes he is experiencing are also significant and he may find that quite enough to deal with without encouraging and supporting you on this front. In this situation, get support wherever you can. Find out about exercise classes and enrol on a course. Seek out other like-minded mothers and take your babies for walks or exercise together. Put together a social network of friends who want to meet, and plan your workout wedge around walking routes to meeting places. Plan enjoyable activities that inspire you and renew your energy when you know your energy levels are lowest. So get organized girl!

'I'm scared I'll leak if I exercise'

Urinary incontinence is very common post-pregnancy, regardless of whether the delivery was by C section or through the birth canal. It affects around 50 per cent of all women and is usually caused by pelvic floor weakness. The pelvic floor muscles (the main one is called the pub-ococcygeous) form a figure of eight shape around the vagina and anus, supporting the contents of the pelvis and abdomen, controlling the emptying of the bladder and bowels and contraction of the vagina. When they become weakened, through misuse, disease or damage, anything from a cough or sneeze to doing a knee lift on the spot can cause urinary leakage.

As soon as possible after delivery, begin Kegel or pelvic floor exercises. Done correctly, they are 90 per cent effective at stopping urinary incontinence. Often, when women say they don't work, it's because they have done too few of them to make a difference, or they've been doing them incorrectly.

- First, you need to identify the right muscles. Sit, stand or lie with your legs apart and your buttocks, abdominals and thighs relaxed. Now pull 'up and in' as if you were trying to stop yourself having a pee (don't actually do this more than once, however, or you may cause a urinary tract infection). Breathing normally, continue to pull up and in through the vagina and the anus. The most common mistakes are to pull in the tummy or clench the buttocks.

Make sure you are doing neither. Once you think you've got the hang of that, try the above exercise in reverse to make sure you can isolate the three stages.

- Now try 'The Lift'. First draw the pelvic floor muscles up the 'first floor' and hold. Still breathing freely, now draw them up further, to the 'second floor'. As you get better at these, you can increase the height of the building and go up to the 3rd or 4th floor!
- Mix both fast and slower contractions for best results and do these exercises as often as you can.

Here are some other tips for alleviating the problem:

- Visit the toilet last thing before you leave the house.
- Don't be tempted to avoid drinking to reduce your chances of an incontinent episode. A small number of people get symptoms of urinary tract infection – such as burning, stinging, and abnormal frequency – when they are dehydrated. This may be because of the concentration of urine or because you have a mild urinary tract infection, which doesn't cause problems when you're well hydrated, but as soon as you become a little dehydrated it flares up. It is essential to keep drinking water to maintain normal hydration.
- Keep caffeine, caffeinated fizzy drinks and alcohol to a minimum if you have a problem – both are diuretics and can cause dehydration.

- Try vaginal weights. These are small weighted cones, which
  you insert into the vagina and then squeeze the vaginal
  walls in order to hold. Ask your GP, community physiother-
  apist or a good pharmacist where you can get these.

'I am simply too tired to make healthy choices'
The fact is you will not be getting enough sleep and even
if you are, it may well be disrupted. If you are getting less
than eight hours of sleep a night you might be contributing to your weight problem. Sleep deprivation disrupts
your body's normal ability to process and control various
weight-related hormones (glucose, cortisol and thyroid
hormones). This imbalance encourages cells to store
excess fat and lowers your body's fat-burning ability. Lack
of sleep may also make it harder to control cravings,
which you will be particularly prone to when nursing a
young baby. However, just nine hours of sleep for three
consecutive nights can reverse this, making weight loss
easier. Here is how to get your zzzzs:

- **Move your body**
  Regular exercise (30 minutes most days of the week)
  reduces stress and raises body temperature, which primes
  you for slumber.
- **Avoid alcohol and food and drink that is high in
  sugar and caffeine**
  These can disrupt your sleep or make it harder to get to
  sleep.

- **Try to set standard bed times and prepare yourself for sleep**

  Try to get to bed at the same time every night and prepare yourself by taking a bath, meditating or listening to relaxing music. Also make sure your bedroom is dark, cool and quiet.

- **Take a siesta**

  When your baby naps you should nap too! If you have endured a sleepless night, take at least a 10-minute nap the next day. It will improve both your mood and your ability to stick to your diet.

'I'm under pressure from my partner to lose weight'

When you already feel the need to lose weight, extra pressure from a loved one can actually make you dig your heels in and not give in to pressure. If you're not in the right space to lose weight, it may only make matters worse. Everybody's relationship is different and when a partner starts telling you to lose weight, you need to quickly establish whether this is going to be constructive to your efforts or destructive. If it's hampering your efforts, don't criticize them, simply ask for a little time and space to sort yourself out or, if it's appropriate, ask for more positive input and support.

'I often indulge in late night bingeing'

Late evening can be a treacherous time for weight watchers – you're tired and, once your baby has gone to bed, you may feel this is the only time you have to yourself. At this time of the day your willpower will be at its lowest and, to make matters worse, research has shown that we naturally want to eat more when it's dark.

So to help ease the urge for night binges, practice the following strategies:

- Don't eat in front of the TV with all the lights out. Turn on all the lights and focus on what you're eating. If you're more conscious of what you are doing you're less likely to succumb to temptation.
- In the summer months, opt to eat outside as much as possible – the longer summer evenings will keep you focussed on the task at hand.
- Drop the baggy look. Don't change into baggy, comfy clothes as soon as the baby has gone to bed. This will only serve to help you forget about your body and stop you from feeling when your tummy has expanded as a result of eating too much. In addition, your man will get used to you looking shapeless and will not be able to compliment you as you change shape – and yes he will notice you changing shape if you follow this plan! Constantly wearing baggy clothes encourages tummy muscles that are already extended to stay relaxed and lazy. Close-fitting clothes will give you a reference point to work with. Take a look at section one, step 1 for more thoughts on elasticated waist bands.

'I feel stressed and out of control'

Being responsible for another life is a big thing and you may feel that you are no longer master of your own destiny. This can lead to feelings of powerlessness and anxiety, as well as putting practical restrictions on the time available to exercise or practice good nutrition. However, it is essential that you build in some time for yourself during these first few months of motherhood, in order to prevent stress building up. Long-term production of cortisol, a stress hormone released by the adrenal glands, has been shown to suppress immunity, which may be why people suffering chronic stress are more likely to get ill. There is also evidence that excessive cortisol release is linked to poor insulin control and a tendency to store, rather than burn, fat as a fuel.

Many forms of exercise, such as yoga, tai chi and Pilates, help to slow the mind and put you back in touch with your body. Alternatively, prolonged, rhythmic activities such as walking or cycling appear to have a calming effect on the mind. You may want to look back at pages 276 and 280 for ideas on exercise and food to suit your mood. Also revisit step 6 in section one to remind yourself of the importance of putting yourself on a pedestal.

It is also a good idea to try and find some time for just you and your partner to enjoy – perhaps a weekend away without the baby. Enjoying activities together will allow you both to recharge your batteries and your relationship.

Fitting in a workout wedge

New mums may have to make do with very small bouts of time in which to exercise. Mini workout wedges, such as those featured on pages 133–145, are perfect for fitting in when baby is sleeping after a feed.

LIFE STAGE

MIDLIFE

You do all the right things – you take the stairs instead of the lift, you walk up escalators, you choose skimmed milk – but somehow, the pounds appear to be creeping on. Many people find, once they reach their mid to late 30s and early 40s, that their healthy lifestyle doesn't have quite the same effect on their waistline as it once did. And although you may be trying to be active and healthy, you feel as if your body hasn't quite got the message.

So what's going on? Well, it's partly an age thing. Although you've hardly even reached middle-age, your body is already beginning to put its feet up. This is compounded by lifestyle factors – you tend to eat out more and your social life becomes less active (no dancing till dawn when you've got a young family to contend with, or a presentation to deliver the next day). Greater affluence tends to bring with it more labour-saving devices and a reliance on driving everywhere, rather than walking or using public transport.

These factors are compounded by the fact that when you cook, it's not just for you but for partner, kids or family – so what *you* want to eat may become overshadowed by others' needs. Add to that the fact that you are always busy and it can feel like you are at the bottom of the priority list.

WHAT'S HAPPENING INSIDE YOUR BODY

From as early as your mid to late 20s, your metabolic rate begins to decline by 2–5 per cent per decade. Muscle mass – the amount of lean, as opposed to fat, tissue you have in your body – also begins to decline. Research suggests that we lose 5–7lbs of muscle mass each decade, causing a decline in daily energy expenditure of approximately 225–300 calories. Factor in the usual drop in activity levels and it's easy to see why we may become not just wiser with age, but wider too!

Fascinating new research shows that stress – often present in bucket loads at this time of life – can also have a serious impact on our waistlines. Dr Pamela Peeke, a researcher at the National Institute of Health in America, has spent many years looking at the link between stress and weight gain and has found that hormonal shifts may be to blame. Emotional stimuli trigger the adrenal glands to pump out adrenaline and cortisol: adrenaline primes the nervous system for action, while cortisol stimulates the release of glucose to provide fuel for the impending 'fight or flight'. Normally, once the crisis is over, adrenaline disperses, but cortisol lingers in the blood in order to stimulate appetite and encourage you to replenish used fuel stores. However, since modern day stresses very rarely result in an actual physical fight or flight response, fuel stores are not depleted and hence the cortisol-induced surge in appetite results in us piling on excess pounds.

DAS MANAGEMENT FOR MIDLIFE

'My life is too stressful and I'm getting thicker around the middle'
As mentioned above, stress can have a serious effect on our waistlines. High levels of stress hormones increase insulin levels, leading to weight gain around the waist. The problem is that intra-abdominal fat, also known as visceral fat, is more metabolically active than that stored on the hips and thighs. While that means it's easier to shift, it also means that continuous loads of fatty metabolites are more easily dumped into the liver's circulatory system, affecting its ability to process sugars and compromising cardiovascular health.

However, even if your life is stressful, all is not lost. Physical activity helps to clear the stress hormones from the bloodstream, while the release of endorphins assists in neutralizing their effects. Research also shows that people who work out have a smaller 'stress response' than those who are less physically active. In studies where people were exposed to extreme cold or loud noises, those who had run a few hours before the ordeal were less stressed by the experience than those who had been resting.

Avoiding high GI foods, which release sugar into the bloodstream very quickly, can also help combat stress fat. Go back to section two, page 86 and read about glycaemic loading. Abiding by the Carb Curfew will also minimize stress-induced overeating.

'I spend all day sitting down'
If your job requires you to sit down all day then you need to compensate for this out of work hours. If you keep yourself fit when you can then you'll counteract the effects of a sedentary job. And if you're highly active out of work hours you'll find you acquire a higher resting metabolic rate – which means you'll be burning more calories, even when you're sitting down!

Even if you are mostly desk-bound, try these strategies to inject a little activity into your day:

- Use the stairs instead of the lift. Just 10 minutes climbing (approximately four trips a day) burns 100 calories and tones up your legs and bum.
- Don't email back, visit your colleagues on foot – you'll burn more than twice the number of calories per minute. Get up and walk for just 5 minutes out of every working hour and you'll have done 40 minutes by the end of the day.
- Make your phone calls standing up, rising up on to your toes a few times to strengthen the calves and boost circulation.

- Shop on foot. Carrying the bags will firm up your upper back, arms and shoulders, and you'll burn the equivalent of a Mr Kipling Bakewell Slice in the half hour it takes to stock up.

Does this tickle your G spot?

Eating just 100 calories fewer per day – the equivalent to a chocolate biscuit or three bites of a burger – could prevent the two pounds that the average person puts on every year, according to research in the journal *Science*. It might not be enough to help facilitate weight loss, say the researchers, but it could halt weight gain.

'My metabolism is on a go-slow!'

One of the key defences against a slowing metabolism is resistance exercise. By doing resistance exercise you can increase your muscle mass, which in turn will increase your metabolic rate by demanding more energy on a daily basis (see What's happening inside my body, on page 326). And although muscle weighs more than fat, it is a denser tissue, so it doesn't take up as much space – which is crucial when we're thinking about clothes sizes. There are considerable health benefits to be gained from resistance training, too. It stimulates bone strengthening, improves glucose metabolism and is associated with better posture and a lower incidence of back pain. There is also emerging evidence that resistance training can help lower resting blood pressure.

Check out page 133 in section two for a strength workout wedge and be sure to include one every week.

Does this tickle your G spot?

It's not just your muscles that grow as a result of regular strength training. Women who work out with weights tend to increase their self-esteem and their body image, too.

'I keep meaning to get a grip, but I never seem to get round to it'
Time may be of the essence at this busy time in your life, but remember, a healthy lifestyle isn't just about taking time, it's about making time too. You may need to re-examine your mindset − if healthy eating and exercise keep taking a back seat, it may be because you don't value yourself enough. Go back to step 6 in section one to remind yourself that your needs are important. You may also find step 3 useful − as it's all about learning to think, say and do as one. Are you establishing and acting in the here and now?

You don't need to spend hours at it to benefit from physical activity − just 10 minutes of moderate aerobic exercise can reduce feelings of fatigue and improve mood. So there's no need to plan an all-out assault on the gym, instead begin by fitting small amounts of exercise into your everyday activity and you'll find it soon starts to snowball.

'I eat when I'm stressed out'
As we learned earlier, moderate aerobic exercise could help to disperse the stress hormones that accumulate in the body, preventing you from feeling compelled to eat everything in sight. Learning how to mitigate your own stress response is also important. For some, it might be something social like an aerobics class or a game of golf (although be warned, a recent study found that stress levels went up in people playing competitive sports if they were very focussed on winning). For others, something solitary, like a long walk or bike ride, might do the trick.

Activities such as meditation, reading and gardening can also quieten the mind – it's important to find what works for you and to schedule relaxation time into your life. Go back to section one and look at steps 1, 5 and 6, too.

Finally, ensure you are getting a balanced diet. The B vitamin complex, found in wholegrain cereals, pulses, nuts, eggs and dairy products, is depleted more quickly when you are under stress – so you may want to consider taking a supplement. Also increase your intake of magnesium-rich foods – almonds or sunflower seeds make a quick stress-busting snack.

'*I skip meals when I'm busy*'
Do you get too busy to eat and then find yourself suddenly starving? This is the kind of scenario that leads to overeating, followed by an energy dip and cravings for starchy foods. To avoid falling into this trap, eat regularly and with awareness. You may want to revisit step 1 in section one for some tips. Small frequent meals increase the 'thermogenic effect' on metabolism, so you give your metabolism little 'lifts' throughout the day, rather than overloading it all at once. Eating breakfast continually comes up in research as a common factor among successful dieters – so skip it at your peril.

'*I'm tired all the time*'
Are you getting enough sleep? Lack of sleep not only saps energy levels and can make you feel anxious and depressed, it may also prompt middle-age spread. University of Chicago researchers found that a lack of deep sleep can reduce human growth hormone levels and lead to weight gain. Growth hormone deficiency was associated with increased fat tissue and abdominal obesity, and reduced muscle mass and strength. They also found that, as we age, we are less likely to get adequate quality sleep.

See page 354 for some tips on getting a good night's sleep – this will help you fire on all cylinders and stop your waistline expanding.

Adrenal fatigue

Do you wake up tired and can't get going until you've had a cup or two of coffee? Do you crave sugary foods, you can't think clearly, you forget things, you come down with any infection going…? If you have all of these symptoms, you're probably convinced you have a serious illness, but it's very possible that you are simply suffering from adrenal burnout. The adrenal glands, situated close to the kidneys, produce not just adrenaline but cortisol and DHEA, a hormone that the body converts into the hormones oestrogen and testosterone. Adrenaline and cortisol are there to help you respond appropriately to daily stress. However, if stress becomes too great – either mental stress or physical stress – then the adrenal glands can become depleted and fail to work efficiently.

Restoring normal adrenal function is possible, but it isn't just a matter of popping a pill or seeing the doctor. Harbouring negative emotions, working or exercising too hard, poor sleep, injury or ill health and poor nutrition all play a role and therefore need to be addressed in order to remedy the situation. Revisit section one – particularly steps 1, 2 and 6 – to examine the possible emotional and psychological factors behind adrenal burnout. Are you feeling put upon? Are you taking on more and more without a thought for yourself? Are you feeling guilty or angry about an unresolved issue?

The following steps will also help normalize adrenal function:

- Go to bed earlier. This is better for the adrenal glands than going to bed late and having a lie-in.
- Get a balanced diet with sufficient protein, B vitamins, magnesium and zinc. Following fundamental six in section two will automatically help you achieve this.
- Schedule in down-time – remember it's not selfish, it's about self care. Check out section one page 60 for a little extra help on this one if you need it.
- Ensure you get physical contact with others every day – even stroking a pet can be beneficial.

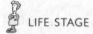 LIFE STAGE

PERIMENOPAUSE

Perimenopause isn't so much a life stage as a pre-menopause stage. Technically defined as the 2–8 years preceding the menopause until one year after your final period, it signals the sharp decline in a woman's fertility and is accompanied by a number of hormonal shifts that can directly and indirectly affect body weight and size. For some women, weight gain seems to occur even when regular exercise and diet are maintained, while, for others, negative feelings about growing older and body image can hamper positive action.

WHAT'S HAPPENING INSIDE YOUR BODY

While perimenopause doesn't normally start until the mid to late 40s, subtle changes in hormones can begin as early as your 30s. For example, levels of DHEA, a hormone that the body can convert into oestrogen or testosterone, decline from the third decade, taking as much as a 50 per cent dive as women approach the menopause. Levels of the appetite-influencing hormone leptin may also fluctuate widely during perimenopause.

From around the age of 40, the body's supply of eggs

dwindles and levels of oestrogen begin to fall. Eggs mature in a more haphazard fashion, causing irregular periods and monthly cycles of differing lengths. These are often accompanied by mood swings and headaches, symptoms that are thought to be due to hormonal imbalances. This can continue for some time, until the supply of eggs runs out completely and periods stop. Many of the symptoms associated with the menopause itself, such as hot flushes, also begin in perimenopause.

As we age, physiological and metabolic processes slow down, often resulting in weight gain – the average woman, for instance, gains 20 pounds between the ages of 20 and 65. However, the good news is that this isn't all an inevitable facet of ageing. In fact, the innate reduction in metabolism and lower aerobic ability is now thought to be a consequence of increasing sedentary living as we get older, rather than an unchangeable physiological process. This means you can do something about it!

By increasing the amount of muscle you have, and reducing the amount of body fat, you can offset this decline and maintain a stable weight. One pound of muscle needs to be supplied with approximately 35–45 calories a day to maintain it, while a pound of fat only demands 2–3 calories. The more muscle you have, then, the more calories you need – and the easier it is to prevent weight gain. (That's why exercise is as important in the Drop a Size plan as nutritional strategies.)

Metabolic Syndrome

Metabolic Syndrome – or Syndrome X, as it is sometimes called – refers to a cluster of symptoms, including high blood sugar, high blood pressure, high levels of triglyceride blood fats and low levels of HDL, the so-called good cholesterol. A high proportion of abdominal fat and large waist circumference are also classic symptoms. Research shows that women who are classified as having Metabolic Syndrome are at greater risk of suffering a stroke and cardiovascular disease. The suspicion is that many more women have this clustering of symptoms but are unaware of it.

Metabolic Syndrome does increase a person's overall health risks. However, the single most important thing you can do to counteract it is to undertake regular physical activity. This will improve glucose sensitivity, decrease blood pressure and improve the level of triglycerides in the bloodstream. Other simple lifestyle changes – such as stopping smoking and losing excess body fat – can potentially reverse the dangers. Recent research from China also suggests that the supplement Tegreen, a derivative of green tea leaf, can help combat the condition by improving glucose metabolism, altering blood fat balance and enhancing insulin sensitivity.

If you have three or more of the symptoms outlined above, see your doctor for advice.

PERIMENOPAUSE DAS MANAGEMENT

'I feel depressed'
If perimenopausal hormone fluctuations are leaving you feeling depressed, you don't need to wait until your official menopause to benefit from HRT. It can make a substantial difference to how you feel at this stage – do bear in mind, however, that it isn't for everyone. Discuss the pros and cons of HRT with your doctor and think about what is best for you.

'I'm getting hot flushes'
Try eating more soya products, as they contain isoflavones, a type of phytoestrogen that has been shown to reduce hot flushes. Experiment with soya 'dairy' products, as well as checking out the Drop a Size for Life foods on page 250. Other nutrients that may help with general symptoms include:

Flaxseed: Add flaxseed to smoothies or porridge oats to help balance hormones.

Calcium and vitamin D: When oestrogen plummets with the menopause you need to put more 'bone in the bank', so getting plenty of calcium and vitamin D is important.

Black cohosh: This can help reduce the physical symptoms of the perimenopause, while chasteberry can help with irregular bleeding.

LIFE STAGE

THE MENOPAUSE

In physiological terms, the menopause signals the end of reproductive potential – there is no longer enough of the hormones oestrogen and progesterone to facilitate repro-duction. However, for many women, the menopause has far greater significance than a mere biological transition. They view it as the slippery slope towards old age or the passing of femininity and hence see it as a mental and emotional change as much as a physical one. This is a time when training your brain – increasing your mind-body awareness – is imperative. Steps 1 and 2 in section one will be very useful at this time, as they will help you stay in touch with – and remain friends with – your body as it goes through this inevitable life change. Your body is still wonderful and feminine and you need to cherish that relationship as much now as at any other stage in your life.

WHAT'S HAPPENING INSIDE YOUR BODY

Menopause normally occurs between the ages of 45 and 55 – the average is 52. The symptoms associated with the menopause – both physical and mental (such as hot flushes, loss of sex drive, weight gain, memory loss, insomnia and mood disturbances) – are commonly put down to hormonal shifts but, in fact, only bone loss, hot flushes and vaginal dryness can be directly attributed to hormones.

One of the most significant physical effects of the menopause is the accompanying detrimental effect on bone density, which is caused by the sharp drop in oestrogen levels (oestrogen plays a role in the deposit of calcium into the bones). Peak bone mass – the maximum amount of bone you ever attain – is achieved around the age of 20 and from the age of 30 or so, bone mass declines by 0.75–1 per cent per year. In the five years following the menopause, bone density can drop as much as 2–5 per cent per year, leaving bones thinner, more fragile and more susceptible to osteoporosis. One in three women over the age of 50 in the UK will suffer an osteoporotic fracture.

Does this tickle your G spot?

Inactive women over 50 are 84 per cent more likely to suffer an osteoporotic fracture than women who do some bone-loading exercise at least twice a week.

RISK FACTORS FOR OSTEOPOROSIS

Early menopause or hysterectomy

Slight build

Family history of the disease

Regular use of corticosteroid drugs

Low lifelong level of weight-bearing physical activity

Low calcium intake

Excessive alcohol or caffeine intake

Smoking

Does this tickle your G spot?

Regular moderate exercise can reduce levels of abdominal fat and shed pounds beyond the menopause, suggests a recent study. Previously sedentary women who cycled or walked five days a week lost 3–7 per cent abdominal fat (which is linked with heart disease and type 2 diabetes) in a year and shed three pounds of body weight. The exact amount lost was proportional to the amount of exercise they performed – the more, the better.

DAS MANAGEMENT FOR THE MENOPAUSE

'Surely exercise will be bad for my bones?'

It's easy to think that if you haven't been active by now, it's too late. Not true! It's never too late and although the 'window of opportunity' for bone building has now passed, weight-bearing exercise can still have a protective effect against further loss. Exercise also improves balance and coordination, which reduces the risk of falls and subsequent fractures. The best kind of exercise for your bones is weight-bearing – so although swimming and cycling are great in some ways, they aren't helpful in this instance. Something that involves you carrying your own weight, such as step aerobics, dancing or jogging, is more beneficial. Another pay-off, as far as your joints are concerned, is that regular exercise can protect against osteoarthritis by keeping joints and connective tissue strong and mobile. Exercise also increases the supply of blood around the joint, thus providing it with a good supply of nutrients – and these, of course, help keep the joint healthy.

Does this tickle your G spot?
Research shows that running has a protective effect against hip fracture, the most common site of fracture in post-menopausal women. One study, which looked at over 4000 women, found that bone density in the femur (the thigh bone) was five per cent higher in joggers than in non-joggers and eight per cent higher compared with those who were complete couch potatoes.

'My weight is beginning to balloon'
The average woman gains two pounds a year around the time of the menopause – weight gain that is widely blamed on the shift in hormones. However, although researchers believe that plummeting oestrogen levels affect the way fat is stored in the body (unfortunately, it encourages an 'apple' rather than a 'pear' shape), it isn't proven that this influences the amount of fat stored. It is more likely that the loss of muscle mass and the accompanying decrease in metabolism is the culprit. This means that by increasing physical activity – both aerobic exercise and resistance training – weight gain can be avoided. Combine exercise with a low-fat, reduced-calorie diet and there is no reason why middle age spread cannot be tackled – it is not an inevitable part of the menopause.

A recent study from Switzerland found that active women in the 55–64 age group gained less than a quarter of the amount of body fat compared to inactive people over a 30-year period. So while you can't expect the same performance from your body at 60 as you could at 30, there's no reason why you shouldn't be able to maintain a close approximation of your ideal body shape for life.

Does this tickle your G spot?
Research on 1,600 women found that physically active women were half as likely to experience hot flushes as sedentary women – yet another reason to get those trainers on.

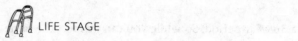 LIFE STAGE

GROWING OLDER

You are in the golden years of life, an era when – theoretically! – you have more time on your hands. The idyllic image of baking biscuits for your grandchildren as they play outside on the lawn, may or may not have come to fruition, but while this time is epitomized as an age when you have time to kick your heels and enjoy your new-found freedom, many people experience depression and a lack of physical confidence as their body changes.

However, don't let what could be described as the autumn of your days become your winter – autumn can be a wonderful and fulfilling time. So instead of setting off on the path of inactivity and speedy ageing, put your DAS maintenance plan into action. Exercise does not have to be vigorous, and healthy eating needn't be extreme, but a little thought and effort means you are investing in your health and putting yourself back in control of your body.

WHAT'S HAPPENING INSIDE YOUR BODY

At this time, your body is experiencing the normal effects of ageing. Everyday activities can become somewhat harder as your aerobic capacity, your reaction time, your muscle mass, your strength and endurance, and your bone mass and density all decrease. So this is a time, more than any other, when exercise should nurture rather than punish your body. It's still great to have goals but don't force yourself to extremes.

The risk of disease is elevated as we age, but one of the single most influential factors is body composition. Excess body fat can, for instance, promote the growth of cancer cells by raising blood insulin levels. In addition, if you are overweight at this stage of your life you can anticipate a higher risk of diabetes and heart disease. But of course, it's not all bad news. Regular, moderate exercise can lower the risk of heart disease among older women by boosting aerobic fitness and trimming tummy fat. One study found that postmenopausal women who began an exercise program of brisk walking or cycling five days a week lowered abdominal fat levels by about six per cent and lost weight overall. Women who exercised for 3 hours 15 minutes a week lost about seven per cent of intra-abdominal fat, compared to those who exercised less than 2 hours 15 minutes a week, who lost just over three per cent. Other recent research found that, for women over 65, increased physical activity still pays dividends in terms of reduced mortality.

> **Does this tickle your G spot?**
> Losing just two pounds is associated with a one per cent
> reduction in cholesterol and a two per cent reduction in
> triglycerides, a type of body fat associated with heart dis-
> ease. It also reduces fasting blood sugar levels, a factor in
> diabetes.

EXERCISING IN THE GOLDEN YEARS

As you get older, the following guidelines will help you
exercise more safely and comfortably:

- Warm up and cool down for longer. Your body will
  naturally take a little longer to warm up and cool down.
  Respect your body and allow 8–10 minutes of gentle
  movement to increase your muscle temperature and keep
  your joints mobile.
- Drink plenty of water. Remember this needs to be little
  and often. Drinking a lot all in one go will put extra strain
  on your kidneys and be less efficient at hydrating you. If
  you are concerned about needing to go to the toilet, get a
  proportion of your water by eating more water-packed
  foods such as cucumbers, radishes, tomatoes, soups, juices
  and milk puddings.
- Be more vigilant when you exercise in extreme heat or
  cold. We get more prone to dehydration and heatstroke
  as we age, therefore very cold weather causes the blood
  vessels to constrict, putting extra strain on the heart.

Dress appropriately for the conditions and allow yourself longer to recover between sessions.

- Ensure you get at least 1000mg of calcium per day. If you take a supplement, look for calcium carbonate with vitamin D (which aids absorption) as more of the calcium is 'available' than from other forms.

A little goes a long way ...

You don't need to be dripping with sweat and panting for breath to reap the benefits of exercise. Nor is there any 'set' intensity that you need to work at for exercise to be beneficial. As long as the pace you set feels at least slightly challenging to *you*, it will be effective in reducing your risk of heart disease.

DAS MANAGEMENT PLAN FOR GROWING OLDER

Your strategy now is to invest in your health. Applying the DAS plan has always been about improving your health but at this stage it may just seem a little more obvious. Besides, you're probably not interested any more in getting into a teeny-weeny polka-dot bikini – but you most definitely want to enjoy spending time with your grandchildren without feeling exhausted. You can add quality and quantity to your years by following the tips in this section.

WARNING SIGNS – GROWING OLDER

You	Warning Sign
I've never been small so what's the point in worrying about it now?	This may be the case but the simple fact is that it's never too late to start. Studies have shown that being active in your younger days and not continuing to be active through your later years provides no protection against heart disease. So stop thinking about exercise as merely a way to control your weight and instead invest in physical activity for the sake of your health.
Carrying a little extra weight is natural at my age	Yes, carrying a little extra weight is natural as your metabolism has slowed down due to the loss of essential muscle mass, but carrying too much will still make you more susceptible to unstable blood glucose and triglycerides.
All that vigorous exercise is not for me	And you are right, vigorous exercise is not right for you at this stage of your life – but moving your body most definitely is. Your body is designed to move so engage in activities that involve more gentle movements, together with co-ordination and balance.
I've never exercised at all and the idea of starting now terrifies me	There's absolutely nothing to be apprehensive about. Think of exercise as movement and medicine for your body and mind.

Action

You need to revisit section one, step 7 and find a G spot relevant to your health. If through your life you have used exercise and diet to satisfy a small spot you need to shift your emphasis and start thinking about adding quality and quantity to your years right now.

You're right up that river – the De-nile! Stop right now and start sailing back down the other way. You need to go back and re-visit step 4 and put your health at the top of your priority list. Don't use the fact that you can be excused for carrying a little extra weight as a reason for not taking action.

Go back to section one and look at it this time with regard to how exercise and physical movement builds confidence and keeps you mentally alert. Enrolling in group activity can provide an important social outlet as well – think about tai chi, organized walking groups, ballroom dancing and yoga.

Get back to training your brain. You need to establish that connection with your body and brain – don't let your body make you look older or feel older than you are.

'My confidence has taken a few knocks'
Your social life may have changed a lot – for instance, you
may have lost a partner or friends – and you may feel you
lack confidence about venturing into new environments.
However, trying new activities and the social interaction
this involves is an important way of building self-esteem
and warding off loneliness.

While physical activity is known to have a positive
effect on depression, you will need to motivate yourself to
get up and out to beat it. The advice in the following chart
should help motivate you.

'My weight gain is down to my thyroid'
Many women at this stage will blame their inability to get
their bodies in shape down, on their thyroid. If you are
exercising and eating your fruit and veg, but you are still
not able to shift the weight, don't just blame your thyroid
– instead, look at the other troubleshooting areas on page
252. The thyroid gland in the neck pumps hormones to
control metabolism and as many as 15 per cent of the
adult population (mostly female) has some degree of
thyroid dysfunction. However, endocrinologists at Miami
School of Medicine estimate only one per cent can claim
weight gain as a direct result. Researchers believe it is
more likely to be a slow gain of 10 pounds that has accu-
mulated over 10 years and gradually comes off when
someone starts thyroid medication. If the weight does not
come off as a result of the medication, then it is unlikely

that the weight was related to the thyroid problem. If you suspect you have an underactive thyroid, called hypothyroidism (other symptoms include fatigue, constipation, muscle aches and cold sensations), or you're frustrated about your weight, your doctor can do a simple blood test to check your thyroid levels.

'I feel I can justify a blow-out at dinnertime'
As we get older, there is a tendency to feel that since your social life is now less important, the simple things in life, like eating and drinking, take on more importance. This, however, is not an excuse to overeat or eat inappropriately. Avoid being lulled into a false sense of security about what you eat. Yes, your nutrition and health has been shaped right through your life but one-off blow-outs such as Sunday roasts, Christmas and holidays are not good for your immediate health, as well as piling on unwanted pounds.

Researchers at Tufts University recommend a nutritional intake for the 70 plus age group of 1200–1600 calories per day. This represents a calorie decrease of approximately 400–800 calories on what is recommended for the younger years of our lives. For this reason it's particularly important that nutrient-dense, rather than high-calorie food is favoured.

So enjoy your food but think about it as a source of health, as well as enjoyment.

Does this tickle your G spot?

Before you indulge in a blow-out meal, think about the following. After just one high fat meal, your arteries may lose 18 per cent of their capacity to expand and contract for the next 5 hours, putting you into what some doctors call the heart attack danger zone – now doesn't that make you think twice about that second helping!

'I can't sleep at night, so I snack'

Many people report experiencing sleeping difficulties as they get older. Lack of sleep at night can leave you feeling tired and disorientated the following day, which in turn can affect your desire to be more active. Many women resort to a sleeping pill to help them get a good nights' sleep and some of these medications can leave you feeling a little drowsy the next morning. In addition, averaging four hours of sleep a night has been shown to increase your risk of type 2 diabetes.

If you do find yourself lying awake for hours, getting up and having a small snack can actually help you get back to sleep. The theory behind this is that when you eat, your metabolic rate increases and your body temperature does too, making sleep easier. This effect is enhanced if you eat snacks that stimulate serotonin release (for instance, a bagel and honey, toast and marmalade or jam, or milk and a digestive biscuit). Serotonin is a brain transmitter that makes you feel more calm and lethargic, making it easier to fall asleep. Having a snack in the middle of the night in this situation is not burdening the body with extra calories, provided you don't eat too much – see the list of 100-calorie snacks on page 194.

You may also need to address the stressful situations in your life that are causing you sleepless nights.

Case Study: Mary's Story

Mary cared for her husband, who had suffered a stroke three years ago. She didn't like taking a sleeping tablet, particularly as she was conscious that her husband would often call out for her in the night. She often had to get up in the night to care for her husband and at such times she found it hard to get back to sleep. On these occasions she would take a sleeping pill but would end up feeling far more exhausted the following day. The sleeping difficulty here was partly induced by stress but by allowing herself some time out – she joined a local walking group – she gained an important social outlet and a diversion from the strain of constant caring. It also improved her physical stamina, too. Mary found that on the nights after she had been out walking, she slept much better, even if she had to get up in the middle of the night to care for her husband.

'I'm too old to change my eating habits!'
It's never too late to start looking after yourself. As we age, the digestive tract can become sluggish so eating foods that provide fibre is important, as is getting plenty of nutrients. So ensure you get a good supply of both. Also be aware of gradual weight gain. In this battle, small simple actions can be the most effective. Even if you eat just 100 calories a day over your target, in the course of a year you could gain 10 pounds. So why not start by cutting your calories by 100 a day and aim to build up your physical movement.

TRY PURÉE POWER!

If you find it difficult to digest high-fibre foods and whole grains, purée can take the place of high-fibre ingredients. As well as providing a great flavour burst, it will give you a fantastic nutrient boost and it's easily digested.

Garlic purée: simmer 1 bulb of garlic in water for 10 minutes. Remove the cloves and purée in a food processor with 2 tablespoons of the water used to simmer it. Store in a sealed container in the fridge.

Leek purée: Simmer the sliced white portions from 1lb of leeks in water for 5 minutes. Purée with no added water and add a pinch of sea salt. Tip – add yoghurt or low fat milk to make excellent bases for sauces and marinades.

White bean purée: Purée white beans with lemon peel and fresh herbs for a high-protein, virtually fat-free dip. Add a little olive oil to boost the benefits to your heart.

SO THERE YOU HAVE IT ...

Dropping a size for life is about finding that relationship with your body that you feel happy with.

You have the tools to make this investment for your health and your body in your hands. Of course, the big issue is motivation and getting in the right mindset to make it happen. Remember, it's okay if your motivation strays – that's natural. That's why I wrote Section One, so you can go back and focus on raising your self-esteem, getting the right mindset and finding that G-spot! Falling back into the rut of one-night-stand dieting won't help you to keep that size off for life, and most definitely won't improve your health. Remember, one-night-stands never deliver the goods in the long term.

Flick back through the Fundamentals and make this part of your day-to-day life. If nothing else, implement my Carb Curfew – it fits in with your life and it delivers results.

Your body naturally changes as you go through life – so make friends with it. You will be rewarded with good health and a great body shape.

Go on, be active! You know you're worth it.

Be active !

Joanna

BODY BLITZ
Permanent Fat Loss in 5 Simple Steps

Joanna Hall's *Body Blitz* will help you design a diet and fitness program that fits in with your life. This way you can make your own realistic goals – whether you're frazzled with kids, working long hours, or simply leading a jam-packed social life.

Just follow the 5 Steps:

1 Use Joanna's Special Starch Curfew Plan
   Stop eating certain carbohydrates after 5pm to boost your energy and lose weight too.
2 Drink a Minimum of 2 Litres of Water a Day
   This way you'll curb your hunger and enhance your nutrient absorption.
3 Decrease Your Fat Intake
   Eat the right fats and see your own body-fat decrease.
4 Make Time for Exercise
   Learn how to fit activity into your day.
5 Be Consistent – At Least 80% of the Time
   Erratic eating will leave you devoid of energy and prone to putting on the pounds.

Joanna Hall includes a 14-day eating plan, over 25 recipes, and many more ideas for starch-free, low-fat meals and snacks. Her program has been tried and tested by real people with real pressures and their own stories and tips will inspire you to win the war against unwanted fat and lack of energy.

DROP A SIZE IN TWO WEEKS FLAT!

The Quick Fix You're Looking for to Get you into Your Jeans, Your Bikini, or that Little Black Dress

Joanna Hall offers you the quick and healthy way to drop a dress size as well as the solution to long-term weight management so you can look good every day of the year.

- Use the Starch Curfew plan: no carbs after 5pm
- Which carbs to choose and when to eat them
- Exercise to get your rear in gear
- Fantastic, easy recipes
- How to use 'Habit Grooving' to make the plan a way of life

CARB CURFEW

Cut the Carbs after 5pm and Lose Fat Fast!

Joanna Hall's Carb Curfew™ is a highly effective and practical diet and fitness plan. It is flexible to fit with your life, however hectic it is, so that you can maintain your weight loss over the long term.

- How to follow Joanna's Carb Curfew™ plan
- Why you should drink 2 litres of water a day
- Why eating the right fats can help your body lose fat
- How to build activity into your day
- Use the 80-20 rule – be consistent 80% of the time

Using these five steps you can really change your level of fitness. And with the delicious selection of Carb Curfew™ recipes you'll lose weight fast.

Make
www.thorsonselement.com
your online sanctuary

Get online information, inspiration and
guidance to help you on the path to physical
and spiritual well-being. Drawing on the integrity
and vision of our authors and titles, and with
health advice, articles, astrology, tarot, a
meditation zone, author interviews and events
listings, www.thorsonselement.com is a great
alternative to help create space and peace
in our lives.

So if you've always wondered about practising
yoga, following an allergy-free diet, using the
tarot or getting a life coach, we can point you
in the right direction.

www.thorsonselement.com

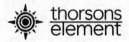

thorsons
element